Orgasm Matters

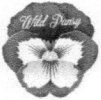

Armin Lear Press
825 Wildlife
Estes Park, CO 80517

ISBN: 978-1-7362988-6-2

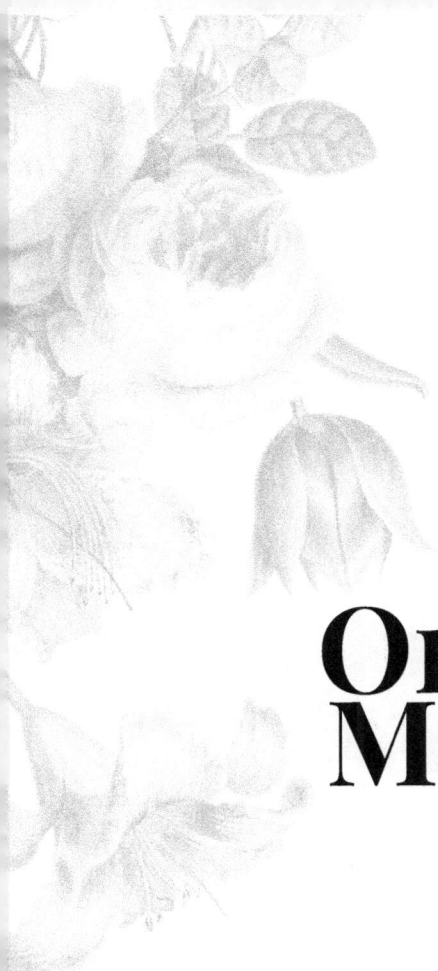

Orgasm Matters

Steven Bodansky, PhD

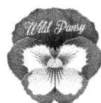

For Vera
My Muse My Mojo My Magic

Contents

Author's Note on Pronouns

This book is for all couples, but the primary emphasis on women and women's pleasure. For that reason, I recommend it primarily for heterosexual couples and lesbians. A lot of information would be useful to gay men, but this is probably not your main book on sexual pleasure—except for the in-depth discussions on communication and prolonging male orgasm.

As for the pronouns, I try to use "he" and "she" when referring to experiences specifically associated with penis and clitoris or vagina. However, I often use "they" to refer to a singular person because the individual could be he, or she, or any gender preference. In short, don't judge my choice of pronouns. Enjoy the information and use it to enhance your pleasure no matter if it involves he, she, or them.

Introduction

This is a book about not only the physical aspects of orgasm but about the process of being present mentally and spiritually with orgasm. I will get you coming and going. The potential to feel orgasmic is available to anyone at any time. Seems like a fantastic claim but I will back it up with the rest of this manuscript. I probably grabbed your attention with those words, although you probably are still not feeling orgasmic. Keep reading if you have the desire to feel it. All you have to do is to notice "it" because "it" is always there. It is there if you can observe it. You can plug into it at any time. It does take some discipline to do this, especially at first, because of where a person's attention usually turns. That is what is getting in the way: the constant thinking and stream of consciousness, or rather stream of unconscious thoughts, that are running through and cluttering your mind nearly all the time.

Putting your full attention on your body, specifically your genitals, in a positive and affirmative way will translate into orgasmic sensation and pleasure. A lot of the work described here (if you can call it work) is specific techniques that will take your potential orgasm and raise it to a more intense level. The ability to just notice your body and have it feel way pleasurable is a great first step on a journey into an orgasmic filled life situation. That does not mean that you will always want to be feeling orgasmic, but it is a lot simpler and easier than most folks think. The times that you desire to, you will be able to.

Orgasm is being conscious of the pleasure that our bodies can feel. You can also have an orgasm and not be conscious, or have an orgasm that is not totally pleasurable. Of course, you can also have pleasure and have it not be orgasmic. The orgasm that I will be discussing in these pages is of the conscious and pleasurable kind—probably the highest form of pleasure that a human being can feel.

The double entendre of the title of this book *Orgasm Matters* is perfect for what we will be considering here. The matters that will be studied are subjects and sub-subjects that have been the focus of much of my adult life situation. I don't use the term "my life" anymore after reading and rereading Eckhart Tolle's works, which I thoroughly recommend. According to Tolle, and I agree, we do not have a life— we are life. We do have life situations however and orgasm has taken center stage in mine. So being that I am under the influence of Tolle and other spiritual masters, I would like to point out here that the words that you will be reading are not *the* orgasm but point to the orgasm. You still will be responsible for feeling it.

It is not just my own orgasm that has entertained my fancy over the years but those of my wife, Vera, and all the students who have come into my life. After all my years of studying and producing orgasms it still fascinates me. Vera fascinates me. I have written her many love poems, each year of the nearly four decades we have been married.

Everyone has some similarities in how they have an orgasm but the differences in the way that diverse women can experience this phenomenon are phenomenal. Men too have differences in how they feel pleasure, only we have not studied that subject to the same diligent extent. For example, some women can only get off on a light stroke, others only with a firm stroke. Some women can only get off with the aid of a vibrator or only by lying on their belly and humping a pillow and others don't require any touching at all. Some women like Vera have strong abdominal ridging where their whole pelvis is undulating and they feel it all over their body from their head to their toes and even beyond their physical body. Many women especially those who have not allowed themselves to explore their bodies have a more localized response, if at all.

One can objectively notice which orgasm is stronger or more intense than another, but the actual pleasure that the person is feeling is subjective. It is not always so simple to say who is having more fun even though the orgasm may seem more powerful in one person versus another. It does seem to be true that everyone is able to improve his or her abilities to feel pleasure and experience longer and more intense orgasms with practice.

I have written comprehensively on the orgasmic subject for years, yet it seems not thoroughly enough as people still have questions that I feel we may have not covered fully in previous works. That is the reason for this book. Plus, I really get a kick out of writing about this topic. We used to have the expression, "The course is for the teachers." The same goes here. "The words written are for the writer."

The first chapter in this manuscript is about you guessed it, orgasm. I go into some detail about the different concepts of orgasm and how one can have one instantaneously. I compare the many types of orgasms and the differences between female and male responses. I describe how to divvy up the roles so that one person is totally having their attention on receiving pleasure and their partner is totally focused on giving them pleasure. In order to give someone authentic pleasure, you have to enjoy what you are doing. I also relate how our work is about manual stimulation and the reasons for that.

Even though our expertise is about manual stimulation we get a lot of questions from women on having more fun with intercourse. The second chapter titled *Healthy Sex* answers those questions as we provide specific information about how women can enjoy intercourse more and what their partners can do to facilitate this. This chapter also includes a section about orgasm in relation to health, both the pros and some of the cons and my personal views on this topic.

I have included in this book a section on self-pleasuring. It is vitally important to know your own body. Then you can communicate your preferences to your partner. If you don't have a partner you still will be able to have a fantastic time. This chapter describes some wonderful techniques to having a party with your pleasure for both men and women, including putting on the lubrication and things that you can do with both hands. I have included a detailed recipe on how to connect your nervous system so that you can have more of a full body orgasm as opposed to just the genitals. There is also information here on connecting the sounds emanating from your throat to your orgasm. There is also a section on fantasy, which is further explored throughout the book.

In the self-pleasure chapter, we have included specific techniques that are unique to each of the two sexes. Just because it is not about self-pleasuring your type of genitals does not mean that you should skip that section. The more that you know about your partner's body and what feels good to them will be beneficial to you in becoming a better lover. Although our expertise is the female orgasm and we write mostly about that, men can benefit appreciably from understanding and applying some of that information to themselves. One time a good friend of ours said, "I'm coming like a woman." His wife said, "Actually you are coming like a person." In other words, guys can learn a lot from how women can experience an extended orgasm and learn how to relax their body and be present with the sensation. We have had both gays and lesbians as our students and a number of them were top-notch researchers.

The fourth chapter is a detailed description on *Overcoming Resistances* and seducing your partner to being done with manual stimulation. Everyone supposedly wants pleasure yet it often remains allusive. Why then do people often say no to pleasure, especially women? There are a multitude of reasons and I think that we have covered most of them or at least many of them here. In this chapter I have described many of the resistances to pleasure that a person may have and how to seduce them into moving into their pleasure instead of having it blocked. It is mostly about how to seduce a woman to have pleasure, but men also resist and this chapter will give you some valuable ideas on ways that you can have fun with resistances.

In order to have a great sex life, to be an amazing lover, a person has to be able to be a responsible communicator. This chapter on *Sexual Communications* will give you many tools as to how to get to that place and be that person. Because of the importance of excellent communication skills, it will be integrated throughout this book as well as having its own chapter. This chapter includes a section as to how to extend an orgasm with words. I will also describe how to use your throat with words or even moans to add to your orgasm. This chapter also contains an in-depth section on how to take control of your partner's orgasm so that they can more easily surrender their nervous system to you. I admit that this chapter strays a bit out of the bedroom but to practice good communication skills at all times will be the best foundation you can build to becoming an amazing lover.

I want to meticulously and methodically with as much fun as I can assemble while writing, cover the topics of "doing." I believe I will stimulate the juice in that fruit. There will be quite a bit of information about giving someone an Extended Massive Orgasm (EMO). That is our expertise and there are a lot of pointers that I will be presenting. I will break down *Giving Pleasure* into two chapters. The first one is *Enjoying the Touch* and will include everything but touching the clitoris and the equivalent male erotic zone. The next chapter is called *Touchdown* and the teasing will be over, as we will get to the clitoris and give you all the tools to create the most exquisite orgasmic sensations in your partner.

There are many aspects to employ to give someone pleasure. There are only a few aspects required to receive maximum pleasure. Though there are not that many things to learn to receive a great orgasm one does have to fully embrace each one of those. This chapter that is called *Receiving Pleasure* describes what these characteristics are and how to accomplish them. These include being in the moment, learning your preferences and communicating them, surrendering your nervous system as you become total effect, learning how to relax your body, and appreciating and acknowledging all that you enjoy. I conclude this chapter with a section on how to receive pleasure by choosing the best positioning for you and your partner.

We had more of a specific agenda and order when writing our other sex books. The two EMO books were systematized. They were organized so that each page when read consecutively was actually depicting the orgasmic cycle. It was a model of an orgasm while describing the different aspects of pleasure and orgasm. We increased the intensity gradually, reached a high point then peaked the intensity a number of times and then brought the intensity back down.

Our third orgasm book titled *Instant Orgasm* was also written in a very specific manner. Instead of taking you through one big orgasm we wished to deliberately describe a first stroke mentality over and over. The result was that we kept going up and down throughout the book. The idea was to keep you as present as possible to teach you to feel each stroke with all your attention. This book has similarities to the way I wrote that book but is more of a stream of consciousness attempt to stimulate my brain or mind into giving up some of its ideas and viewpoints on the years that I have been studying orgasm. This may seem like it is too heady with too much thinking. I promise that it will involve a lot of feeling and keep your attention on your pleasure. I want to explore orgasm from different aspects, angles, and viewpoints so that you will be ready to take your pleasure to a new horizon. It will feel at times that you are inside the orgasm perhaps the proper metaphor would be comparing it to being in the eye of a hurricane. We also will be moving out of the eye so brace yourselves for some wild fun.

I find it interesting that when I wrote my first fictional book that I also named *Extended Massive Orgasm: the Novel,* I had frequent orgasms while writing it. I was turned-on by my fantasies and really enjoyed the creative sexual energy that I generated. I have not had the same experience with any of my other non-fiction books except for a couple of times that I was writing this one. I did not have that experience writing my other novel or with writing poetry. It did not make for a better book perhaps but it did make it even more fun to write.

According to Eckhart Tolle there is probably some correlation between how present one is at the time of writing or doing anything for that matter and how beneficial ultimately that piece of work becomes. I just am not sure of the connection between how much joy went into something and how much joy comes out. It would be difficult to measure just as the orgasmic pleasure someone is feeling is subjective.

It also is quite clear that my attention span for writing and sitting down to express my thoughts is limited no matter how much fun it is. I usually sit for between a half hour to an hour when I write, with fortunately most of my attention on what I am writing about. I enjoy the writing process when I am doing it but after that certain length of time I have had enough of writing and lose interest no matter if I am in that orgasmic writing state or not. I also do not like to spend too much time on the computer, as my eyes, knees and back will find a reason to revolt. Even when I am writing a poem with a pen and paper it seems that an hour or so is optimum for my attention span.

When I am writing a non-fiction book like this, my attention is not on my genitals except when I'm describing some fantasy section. Most of the time that I'm writing here I am focused on the thoughts that are triggered by what I have just written. I am more involved with my mind than with my body, opposite to when I was writing the sexy novel. My attention is on my thoughts and what those inspire me to write next. I enjoy the process intently, but I have had enough of that kind of concentration within that span of half an hour to about an hour. I still spent about the same period of time and feel spent when I wrote that novel despite the orgasm energy. It's a combination of not wanting to sit any longer and just feeling spent up for the time being on the process of focusing on generating meaningful words. I think I spent more time per writing session on my first book, which has been the most successful but not the most pleasurable one to write.

I think that I am pretty much the same way with having sex and orgasm in that I am not a marathon runner. I am more of a sprinter or at best a mid-distance candidate. I have done demonstrations on women for an hour but those were special courses designed to show what is possible. I have even done Vera for three hours a number of times because it was part of a course or an assignment. (It's okay to brag once in awhile). A half an hour is usually more than enough time to give or receive terrific orgasmic pleasure. Our sensuality teacher, Dr. Victor Baranco once said that one could fully pleasure a woman in twenty-seven minutes if you know what you are doing. That is almost thirty minutes of orgasm where you are feeling a lot of pleasure from the start. It is not like warming up for twenty minutes and then finally starting to feel good. You are having contractions and all the signs of orgasm from the first few seconds onward.

I think that when a lot of couples hear about extending the orgasm, they will tend to overdo the process, thinking that more and longer is better. It is better perhaps up to a certain point but there is a diminishing return after a while for most people. I am sure there are some marathoners out there who feel differently. I just think that many people do it for the success rather than the pleasure after a certain point. Also if you are not feeling for the first twenty to twenty-five minutes and then you start to feel you will want more time. Learn to start from the get-go and have it all feel wonderful; then you will not feel shortchanged.

I live the same way that I write and have sex, in that I only desire to do things with as much pleasure and fun as I can. This does not mean that everything that comes my way is easy or would sound like fun to everyone. Everybody that I have ever known has been or will be challenged in their lives in some area whether it is relationship, health, finances or whatever. It is how you accept the challenges and how you use them to grow spiritually that can make a difference.

Although this book is about orgasm you will notice that I have also included some intimate and personal information about Vera and me in order to transmit certain matters. I am of the ironic belief that the more that you can expose of who you authentically are, the actual freer you will be. I think that it also creates some affinity between you the reader and me the writer. I therefore decided to include some personal and anecdotal information throughout this book. For several years Vera has been losing her memory, both short term and long term. This has not always been an easy thing to deal with, yet I think because of our training in pleasure and living pleasurably we have been handling it better than I or anyone for that matter would have expected. Vera is just as positive and, if possible, more loving than she has ever been. My practice of daily meditation has also helped, as I feel more patient and loving too. My love for Vera has only grown stronger and fuller. I would say that she is not suffering from her illness; rather she goes with the flow of her life and is in agreement with the way things are instead of fighting the veracity of her situation. Even though she does not remember facts or people she does remember how to love and be loved. I still give her orgasms regularly and have become even more creative in how to get her aroused. A lot of the information in the first *Giving Pleasure* chapter was developed these past few years.

Vera is very dependent on me and surrenders to what I want her to do with as much ease as someone totally in serenity and love. She has her moments of resistance but those are quite rare. She has not forgotten how to be stubborn. I know that in the man/woman relationship the fulfillment of the feminine desire and promise is the loftiest potential that the couple can aspire to. Vera has been a fantastic partner and muse as well as shown me how she prefers to be treated and loved. Even though at times it seems that we are doing what I want or what I say; I believe that we are really doing it her way. Because of her fulfillment our relationship continues to thrive despite the obstacles that we face. I thought that although quite personal our continuing story and challenges has importance for other people with dementia and other disabilities. I have written a book totally dedicated to what we are going though titled *Love and Alzheimer's*. It is ongoing in my blog as well and certainly a joyous one at this moment. I am grateful to the writings of people like Eckhart Tolle and Frank Kinslow who have given me the tools to quiet the mind and enjoy this moment. And orgasm and dark chocolate do play their parts extremely well.

Some of you have been to and seen a live demonstration of a one-hour orgasm either with us or at *Morehouse* or with some of the now various offshoots that have developed over the last few years including our offspring the *Welcomed Consensus* and *One Taste*. We also have a video version for sale that some of you may have watched of Vera having a one-hour orgasm demonstration. Probably most of you however have not had this life-changing opportunity to experience this in person or via the video.

In order to start doing something, for instance having orgasmic pleasure or writing as I am now, it helps if you have enthusiasm in your corner but it is not necessary. Sometimes it is fine to just begin. Just start writing. The same with having an orgasm; it helps but it is not necessary to have extreme passion. Just start talking with sexual interest or about how attracted you are to your partner. Make your partner an offer for fun and at some point, perhaps if you both are willing, with touching them. If you don't have a partner self-pleasure can begin in the same manner. If you like pornography or fantasy you can use that to get in the mood. Otherwise you can create the time and space and just start feeling and playing with your own body. Once you begin the desire will often come along for the ride and take over, as enthusiasm likes to do.

1
Matters of Orgasm

Many things are better done unconsciously than consciously, such as digesting and other bodily processes. Others are best done with your full attention, bringing to bear as much awareness as you are able to manifest. We are only really able to focus on one thing at a time so we may think that we are multitasking, but we are just quickly going back and forth with our selective focus. You cannot be lost in thought and really focused on what you are doing at the same time with any great aptitude.

Conscious, consciousness, and even awareness are not simple words that can be pin-holed into one thing. They have been called suitcase words or words with a variety of meanings. You can fit a lot of different things in them or that they describe a bunch of different things for a bunch of different people. The same can be said for the word orgasm. It can mean different things to different people depending on their viewpoint and how the word is used and understood. Some people have orgasm as the climax of sexual tension, a complete muscular release and lasts for only a few seconds if one is lucky enough to get there.

We see orgasm as the pleasurable sensation that you can start experiencing before even being touched and that continues and grows even stronger as you are touched. By putting your attention specifically on your genitals and on any of your gratifying bodily sensations and approving of such you can easily develop your pleasure intensity. It has been said that your brain (mind) is your largest sex organ. It is definitely the one that will be at the forefront of any pleasurable experience although it can get in the way of the same if you have your attention elsewhere.

Orgasm is there for the noticing. It is not some difficult and arduous task. It is up to you though to become aware of this and selectively notice. When most people have sex they are being very future oriented and trying to get to a certain level with physical sensation and focusing on the goal while actually being unconscious of a lot of what they are actually feeling in the present. To have the optimum orgasmic experience one has to be fully conscious of the sensation that they are involved in. Participants focused on the future are missing the pleasure of now for the hope of some subsequent pleasure. Sensually that just does not make sense.

Men Make Lousy Orgasmic Role Models

Most men in order to have an orgasm will tense up and tense up and tense up and then finally climax. Orgasm over. Men have learned to tense up their bodies to experience orgasm and equate their orgasm to their ejaculation; women have copied this singular behavior as that is all that they have probably witnessed in as far as an orgasm. Sensually speaking one can feel far more in a relaxed state than in a tensed up one. Because of the habit of tensing up that people have developed, the learning to relax to feel more is sometimes a process that may take some practice. You don't have to give up tensing up all together, but we urge you to explore the possibility of what you can feel in a relaxed state. Our work and techniques are based on a person being relaxed and not tensing up. We will get into this topic in further detail later on in the *Receiving Pleasure* chapter and throughout this book.

Is it Pleasure or is it Orgasm?

The line between being in a state of pleasure and being in a state of orgasm is kind of fuzzy for lack of a better word. When does pleasure turn into orgasm? It is probably a subjective experience and as I say hard to pinpoint or a fuzzy line. I know that when I am being pleasured at some point it just feels that I have transcended into a level of pleasure that feels to me orgasmic.

With women who have trained their bodies in orgasmic studies it seems that they can easily cross this line without even being touched. Before I stroke Vera, I can notice that she is already showing some, if not all, signs of orgasm including a wet pussy, contractions and genital engorgement. She was not always able to do that at will, but she was a quick learner and a good student. According to what Vera has told me she has been orgasmic most of her life. She told me that she would even "get off" from the repeated motion on the seats of the wooden trains and trolley cars in Europe after World War II when she was around eleven years old.

I have danced with some orgasmically trained women whom I could tell were having an orgasm while in my arms. I don't think that women have to be even trained to have that kind of experience though they may not realize it as easily as someone who is. Some women have a more difficult time experiencing pleasure this easily. We have found that every person is able to increase their orgasmic energy and their orgasmic capability with some positive attention placed upon this subject. Studying orgasm matters.

The key to having this kind of easily orgasmic experience is to feel your body with as much pleasurable attention as you can muster and not to judge and ponder about whether you are or are not having an orgasm. The goal has to be just the pleasure at this moment. When you jump outside this time frame you are in your head and not feeling your body. The orgasm for surely will come along for the ride but you cannot force it to. The better you are able to stay present and appreciate any pleasurable sensations that you have will create the juice upon which the orgasm flows. All you have to do is to feel, "Yes" to any pleasurable feelings and those feelings will grow. If you think that it is not good enough or think that it should feel otherwise then you are thinking and not feeling.

Short Exercise

Right after reading this paragraph, for a few seconds or so, put this book aside and put your attention on and focus on your genitals. By putting your attention there you will be able to notice them and may feel some pleasure. Approve of any sensation you feel whether it is heat or tingling or perhaps more than that. It is very simple and you don't have to work at it. If you do not feel any sensation at all this first time that is okay, too. No pressure. It is only for a few seconds. You can close your eyes if that helps. You can take a few deep inhale and exhale breaths if that helps but you don't have to. Put the book aside now and begin feeling your pussy (clitoris) or your penis.

Welcome back. Because of the concentration of nerve endings on the clitoris being more numerous and concentrated than on a penis, women may have an easier time with this exercise than men, but other factors will also influence how much you feel. These will include your ability to focus and whether you may have strengthened these nerve pathways previously. The more you repeat this exercise the easier and more you will feel. This is something you can do as a practice for a few seconds at almost any time of the day to develop your focusing and sensitivity. For example, I would love it if you would do this exercise whenever you pick up or put down this book before and after reading it for just a few seconds. You will learn to love this exercise too.

Orgasm Prejudice

It has been thought and expressed that generally men reach orgasm faster than women. This is because folks have been prejudiced by their lack of knowledge on the topic of female orgasm. We have come to the opposite conclusion that it is actually easier for a woman to have an orgasm. For this to be true, she has almost certainly studied her orgasmic potential and has trained to focus on her genitals and specifically on her clitoris. The origin of this prejudice is obvious. Most people are describing what happens to the man and the woman when they are having coitus. It is understandable that the man will have an easier time "reaching" orgasm when it is his most sensitive sex organ that is being stimulated while the woman's most sensitive area is usually being ignored. Fortunately, there is a lot more information now than when I was growing up, which is not that long ago bearing in mind how many centuries female orgasm was not considered or comprehended at all.

There have recently been some studies where men and women were asked to have an orgasm while their brains were being studied with MRIs and Pet Scans. I guarantee that they were self-pleasuring to reach this goal. It was found that men and women's brains were quite similar as to which areas were lit up when having the orgasm. It was not just one centered area that lit up but about thirty different areas throughout the brain; including the area accountable for touch or the sensory cortex, the limbic system that is linked to our emotions and memory, the hypothalamus, which is associated with unconscious body control, and the prefrontal cortex that is correlated with our judgment and thought center.

The female's orgasms lasted for about twenty seconds and the male orgasm lasted for about ten seconds. There were no studies reported on a relaxed extended orgasm, so all of those reported were of the tensed-up variety. A few of the women were even able to have an orgasm without touching themselves but by just thinking about one. Their brains lit up in the exact same way as those who physically touched themselves including the brain area correlated to touch.

Different Types of Orgasm

Some people have either a natural ability or have built a connection between their genitals and other body parts such as their nipples, their facial lips and other sensitive areas on their bodies. They can experience orgasmic sensations when having those regions stimulated without genital stimulation. In the self-pleasure chapter, we will provide you with some key exercises, which will help connect your isolated body parts.

Vera and I and our colleagues were taught that all female orgasm is clitorally based and I have also read where others believe that there are different kinds of orgasm such as clitoral and vaginal. As we learned more about the entire clitoral structure, we discovered that the clitoris is both inside and outside. Regardless of how you refer to the type of orgasm, all varieties studied supposedly all light up the brain similarly.

Is it then the brain or the mind that is the base for all orgasms? Probably the correct answer is a big yes and also a little no. As we have seen the brain lights up when having an orgasm of any kind in similar fashion. On the other hand, I have witnessed women who were having a full body and clitoral orgasm who did not realize what they were feeling. They just could not tell that they were having this experience. They were new to this sensation and unfamiliar with this different feeling of coming when relaxed. They were being unconscious of their body's response. After being exposed to this orgasmic familiarity for a number of times they were able to connect their brains to their pussy and learned to enjoy what their body was going through and had been going through. The nerve pathways become strengthened with repeated experiences. It's kind of like the old Zen question about whether there is any sound if a tree falls in the woods and no one is there to hear it? Eventually someone does if trees continue to fall.

Division of Labor

In our work, we have consistently divided most of our sensual experiences into giver and receiver, or cause and effect. This means that one of the sensual partners will have all of their attention on producing pleasure in their partner's body. The person receiving this pleasure also has their total attention on their own pleasure. For the entirety of this orgasmic act both people keep to their roles. There is no going back and forth as to where the attention is focused. A person can experience the most pleasure when at total effect and all their attention is available for feeling.

When the person has had enough pleasure and is fully done, then they can reciprocate and switch roles or not depending on how both parties feel. This allows for maximum attention on a person's pleasure or orgasm and is recommended for those of you who desire to experience the most pleasure attainable. Both partners are putting their attention on the one orgasm.

You are not required to give up anything that you are already doing that you are enjoying, just to perhaps adding something different to your repertoire. Often when a couple first gets together there is a lot of chemistry that kindles the flames of passion so that you are both feeling the pleasure at the same time. There is a lot of it to go around at the early stage of a passionate relationship. Unfortunately, or fortunately, this passion decreases in most couples over time. The techniques that we espouse will keep the pleasure flames lit over a lifetime. This focusing of one's attention to a particular endeavor or role will enhance your awareness of the experience and make it possible to feel even more when you return to your regular lovemaking.

"Yes! Hands"

Also our work is based primarily on the most efficient way of giving someone orgasmic pleasure which is with their hands to the genitals of their partners. Again, if you enjoy oral stimulation or vaginal penetration with a penis, we are not suggesting that you give those up. Oral stimulation can be erotic, fun and exciting. When a person has not trained to use hands as a sensual tool it may seem to be easier and more fun to do cunnilinguous or fellatio. The fingers however are more precise than your tongue when one learns to use them properly. It is also a lot easier to communicate to your partner when you are not using your mouth elsewhere. When pleasuring a clitoris, the fingers can get to an exact spot with better visualization and preciseness than when using one's tongue. We like to use the analogy; would you want a male brain surgeon doing the surgery with his tongue, penis, or hands?

When stimulating a woman's pussy with my hands for my own pleasure, which is all of the time that I relate with one, I have noticed that I sometimes will feel pleasurable sensation in my own genitals. I will feel myself getting engorged and many of these times I will leak some semen as well. I can feel this happening at times but other times I am not aware of this occurrence until afterwards when I touch myself there or feel some wetness. The pleasure and engorgement in my penis are usually for a percentage of the time that I am stimulating her but can be for a lot longer.

It Must Be Turn-On

I am not sure of the relationship between what the woman is feeling or perhaps thinking and my reaction. The reason I say this is that there does not seem to be a cause and effect response based on how well she is getting off. She can be having a gangbuster fantastic orgasm and I don't feel anything in my crotch, or she can be having a moderate orgasm and I am feeling her very intently there. She can be exquisitely beautiful or not and it does not seem to make a difference to where and how that I am feeling her. Therefore, it probably has to do with her turn-on that is specifically directed *at me*. In addition, it also depends on what she is feeling *about herself* in relation to me or to cock at that time. Our teacher, Dr. Vic Baranco, said and I am just paraphrasing here: "The male human being can feel a woman's turn-on when she is thinking or really feeling in and about her pussy in relationship to cock, specifically whomever she directs it to."

I have noticed that when we talk to our female clients in a session before touching them and have them deliberately put attention on their pussy and clitoris that I can feel it in my genitals, too, when they do so. This can be anywhere from a tingle to a fully erect member depending on how unadulterated their purposeful attention is. It is easy to notice when they are doing a good job of focusing on their pussy and when they are back in their heads thinking about mundane things. It probably also has to do with my ability to focus on my penis, a response probably related to what she is feeling at the time. I specifically request and ask them to feel their pussy and I put my attention on my genitals to determine if they are. Other trained women whom I have worked with can also feel their pussy in response to the student's focus.

In this situation where I am deliberately putting attention on my penis in relationship to the woman feeling her pussy is different than when I am rubbing her. When I am stroking her genitals I am usually focused on my fingers and the engorgement and pleasure in my penis is something that I notice, but it is not something that I am focused on as with the deliberate request and exercise that I just described. My response may also have something to do with whether she is having sexual thoughts in general, sexual thoughts about a penis, or thoughts about my penis specifically.

Orgasm or Just an Arousal Phase?

A student of sexology recently argued with me about whether an extended massive orgasm (EMO) such as the one we profess is an orgasm or not, especially in a male. I agreed that there is emission and ejaculation when a man is being stimulated though the two are not so easily separated. The goal for us is what is most pleasurable, and I believe that the orgasm is not just the ejaculation but also the process that feels the most pleasure. Since a woman does not have to ejaculate to have an orgasm, climax seems to be connected to how tense or relaxed she is in relation to this letting go. It seems that when a woman tenses up and has the climactic orgasm she has had enough for now. She is done. However, the refractory period for some women can be extremely short hence the possibility of multiple orgasms.

A woman who is relaxed while being stimulated can have an orgasmic response of equal or greater intensity to her sister who tenses, only she can continue to feel pleasure; hence the term extended orgasm. The orgasm just keeps on going, although there are peaks of intensity that are in some ways similar to a woman who has multiple orgasms. The level of intensity in an EMO does not come down energetically once she has learned to have this relaxed orgasm in comparison to when she has a tensed up climactic type of orgasm. To us, a woman is orgasmic either way.

It takes a person who has tensed up her whole life and switches to being relaxed a considerable amount of practice to reach the intensity level that she was feeling when she did tense up. Therefore, a lot of our female students will continue to desire that specific sensation. They will tense up their bodies at the end of an extended orgasm. They will continue to do that until they have reached a level of proficiency in intensity with their relaxed orgasmic response.

We have noticed that women who have learned to have a powerful relaxed EMO will no longer have that burning desire to tense up and climax. Some women who have not had either kind of orgasm will still want to have that tensed up orgasmic sensation experienced even though they are learning how to have a relaxed orgasmic pleasure. Why not be able to have it all?

For a male, the point of no return is ejaculating and considered the orgasm. The arousal phase and whether you call it excitement or plateau stages, as Masters and Johnson did, or whatever happens before the ejaculation can be very similar to what a woman is experiencing in an EMO. The man too can learn to relax and feel more and for longer. So yes, there is a difference in sensation between when a male ejaculates or not and, yes, they both feel great. I just feel better usually, but not always, if I don't go over the point of no return and come close to it, but do not have an ejaculation. Sometimes when you are playing on the edge you will go over. My advice is that when you do, enjoy the heck out of it.

There are different levels of intensity that a male can feel just as a female does who is experiencing an extended orgasm. It is difficult to measure how much pleasure objectively a person is feeling. I know that for myself it can feel great just putting on the lubrication or starting to stroke the penis. It can feel really good even if the penis is flaccid. If you are worrying about not being hard you will be having your attention on that thought and not on the pleasure. Just enjoying the touch usually will engorge it and if you want to add a thought add one such as one of your fantasies that increases your pleasure not one that subtracts from it.

Engorgement Matters

Being that we are on the topic of engorgement, unless there is some physical problem with a man's circulatory system such as in diabetes or some other erectile dysfunction, a penis should respond to real female desire or to one's own fantasy and or touch.

There can be a number of reasons why a penis is not getting engorged when a woman claims to want intercourse. The number one cause is that she really does not want it at that moment. She may think that she should, but that has nothing to do with how she really is feeling. She may want some sensual attention, not necessarily intercourse, and wants her partner to overwhelm her with some other form of pleasure. She also may want to play with his penis just not inside her vagina at that moment. She may have doubts about her body and her attractiveness, or she may be too angry with her partner or another person. Anger and doubt will both kill turn-on and destroy any engorgement.

Another possible cause is that he may be responsible for this lack of engorgement himself. The guy may be too concerned with his performance and his thoughts are somehow interfering with his erection. He may have gotten off and even had coitus with another woman recently and his penis is just not ready to respond. He may just find her to be unattractive and is resisting her turn-on. This resistance can only go so far and if she has real desire it will trump any of his resistances. She just may have to turn up her thermostat. He can have his own doubts as he had previously failed or thought that he failed in his last attempt.

The best way to proceed when something like this occurs is to communicate more. If anger is involved, you will have to put your attention on more fun ideas. If doubts are involved, then expressing them will bring you closer to your partner. No one is to blame here. Ask each other questions that show your genuine care and curiosity about one another. You can have fun starting from any situation. Doing her first manually can be a great alternative. A woman ought to be engorged before intercourse just like a man. Perhaps once her juices start flowing freely her desire for intercourse may grow. In any case you have had some fine pleasure.

Male Orgasm

There obviously is some threshold that one crosses when you can say for sure something feels orgasmic rather than just pleasurable. I know that usually at some point I am having multiple contractions and often oozing semen from my penis. This can be at the hand of someone else with a lot of communication or doing it to myself. At what point did the pleasure announce itself as an orgasm? Was it when I noticed the contractions? Probably Masters and Johnson would call all this pleasure the arousal stage, but we believe that it is a real orgasmic experience. By getting close to the edge and backing off and staying in a fairly relaxed state one can peak a man just like a woman only that the ejaculatory point of no return can end this extended ecstasy with just one extra stroke or one little bit of extra sexual thought. The more that I have practiced this technique the better it feels and the more control I seem to demonstrate yet there are times when a sexy thought or a momentary unconscious extra stroke can still send me into an uncontrollable orgasmic ejaculation. At that point, it's time to not fight the inevitable. It would be silly to ruin this fun time with self-reproach.

When I was a lot younger, as with many males it was pleasurable to go for another ejaculation again and again after some short refractory period. This again could be with a partner or with oneself. The older men get the refractory period also gets longer between ejaculations or actually the desire for one. The older and more mature that I have become has made this refractory period longer and longer and the ejaculations less frequent. It is probably true that if one had more than one desirous female partner who wanted a hard penis that this refractory period would be shortened but I have no recent data for myself on this. It probably also would reflect how desirous for a hard penis even a single partner is.

When I was young and probably for most boys orgasm is practiced almost entirely with themselves. The stroking and the ejaculations were pleasurable to some extent. It was basically to release the tension and it also felt good to do it. I did not use any lubricant except maybe saliva when I was first doing it to myself. It was quick and to the point. I usually did it standing up and releasing into the toilet and not making any sounds as it was secretive and I did not even discuss it with my twin brother who otherwise I would tell everything to. There definitely was no trying to extend the pleasure; just get it over with and quickly.

Now after an extended orgasm with many noticeable contractions, I have found that after a while of doing this it just seems to be time to stop. I could go on for another peak and will experiment at times to see if I can extend it some more. It usually seems that I can get back up there again with little trouble. Normally, I will just stop after ten to twenty minutes of orgasmic peaking and consider it enough. I don't usually repeat this extended orgasm more than once in a day, but I do feel that I could do so pleasurably if called upon. I do recall having done so in the not so distant past. It would be a lot more difficult to get it up if I had just had a full ejaculation, though I did that too when I was younger.

Even though we are coaching women to have better orgasms we frequently get questions about stroking a penis. One of the common complaints is that the guys will rub too hard on the woman's clitoris and will want the woman to use a lot of pressure and fast strokes on his penis. The objection is that rubbing on a guy that way is a lot of work for her. To continuously have to do that to her partner and not get a tired or an achy hand is problematic.

I think that when I first started masturbating, I used quite a bit of pressure and fast strokes on myself. Over the years I have learned to like the strokes on my penis to be slower and lighter. The guys who like it hard and fast are used to this and have not trained their bodies to appreciate the more delicate strokes. One of the techniques that we offer these couples is to mix up the peaks by changing the stroke when you change the peak. Talk to each other first so everyone is on board and knows what the plan is. So, one peak you can go hard and fast, another one you can do slow and light. A third peak you can use light pressure but faster and an additional peak you can try hard pressure but go slowly. Guys like to get into a rhythm or pattern and that is why it is a good idea to not keep changing the stroke inside of a peak but to take a break between peaks and then check out a different pattern on the next peak. Women also like a rhythmical pattern. If you keep doing the light and slow stroke over time he will learn to appreciate that too. Just don't give up using the more wearisome fast and firm pattern until he has adapted to enjoying the less tiresome ones. It is also true that you do not want to pleasure someone if it is not fun for you. Only use as much pressure and speed that you can enjoy doing for how long you can enjoy doing it.

Quite a few women prefer to get guys off by fucking them. In some ways it is easier and it takes less attention for the woman to get the guy off that way; and it won't tire out her hands. This can be acceptable to both the woman and the man. However though acceptable and possibly fun we think that it is best if it does not exclusively take the place of a hand job or oral sex. I heard comedian Chris Rock say some funny lines about sex after getting married. It had to do with the same theme of married women no longer giving their husband manual or oral sex and only getting them off by fucking them. Basically, what he was saying is that they fuck their husbands just so they stop pestering them. If a guy can learn to get off with a lighter and easier stroke and if a woman can learn to enjoy herself with her partner's penis is a wonderful recipe for intimacy and a more fun relationship.

2
Healthy Sex

This chapter will cover the ways to improve a female's chances of having an orgasm with intercourse. We will also delve into some of the health benefits known and theorized that orgasm may provide as well as some of the possible negative effects.

Female Orgasm during Intercourse

We get a lot of emails and questions from women about how to have more frequent and better orgasms while having intercourse. It is fairly commonly known these days that a large percentage of women do not have orgasms while engaged in coitus. Even if they do have it occasionally a lot of women do not have it every time.

We recommend that they first learn how to have better orgasms with direct clitoral stimulation. That is something that most women seem quite capable of having except for the small percentage of anorgasmic females. This condition is so rare that we have yet to really experience this in our practice where we have seen roughly thousands of women. We have read about this condition and I suppose anything is possible or not possible. I think society would benefit if teenagers were taught about sexual pleasure and how they could have this pleasure without having to rely on intercourse. An excellent book on that subject is *On Blossoming* (Skyhorse, 2019) by Gia Lynne.

We tell those females who want to experience more pleasure with intercourse to be sure to be engorged before doing it. The clitoris comes in various shapes and sizes and also in different positioning distances from the vaginal opening. "A pussy is like a snowflake. No two are alike; with enough heat they all will melt." (That was a quote I concocted to speak, as one of the lines in our movie role that I will write.) Some women have a very short separation and others have quite a large space between their clitoris and their vaginal opening. When the clitoris is close to the introitus (another word for this opening) it makes it a lot easier for a woman to experience coital orgasm. This is because there is direct contact with her clitoris and his inserted penis. When there is a large space between the two it is more difficult for women to come to orgasm with penile penetration, as her clitoris will not have any direct stimulation.

Engorging the female genitals including the labia and the clitoris before penetration will decrease the length of separation in every woman. The clitoris gets larger and the engorgement appears to move it closer to the opening of the vagina. It is a change of approximately 10 to 35 percent closer in most women with full engorgement. This is enough for some women to have clitoral stimulation with the motions of coitus. Some female clitoral to introital separation is just too great to have their engorgement overcome that gap to an appropriate distance. All the foreplay arousal in the world will not make this distance short enough so that the clitoris would become stimulated with coital penetration. Regardless, being engorged for a woman is just as important to her fun as the male's engorgement.

The other upshot to being engorged and stimulated is that the woman will already be orgasmic and aroused and will feel more in any case. We almost always recommend that it is a good idea to stimulate her clitoris and her genitals to some degree before intercourse. A woman can be wet and still not engorged. It just makes intercourse that much more pleasurable to get her pussy really awakened and aroused before any insertion. The more a woman is enjoying the act will make it that much more fun for the man too.

Connecting the Clitoris to Vaginal Opening

The other technique that we recommend to aid in coital orgasm is to do the connections exercises between the clitoris and the labia and with the introital area. By doing this a woman will generate more sensitivity and feeling in those areas so that she can become orgasmic by just having those areas stimulated and will not have to depend on direct clitoral stimulation with coitus. We will go over in detail in the self-pleasuring section how to build a connection. This can be practiced with one's partner as well. We will give you the fundamentals here.

Here are the essential steps:

- Stimulate the clitoris until it feels good.
- Do the exact same stroke including the same speed, pressure and motion on a secondary area such as the left labia in synchronicity with the stroking continued on the clitoris.
- Stroke on both areas at the same time for a while and then remove the hand from the secondary area and continue stroking the primary area or the clitoris. Keep your hand off but you can leave it almost touching still doing the stroking motion until the sensation subsides.
- Then put your hand back and rub both areas simultaneously again.
- Next time, take your hand off the clitoris and keep stroking the secondary area. Keep doing this back and forth, stroking between the primary and the secondary areas and stroking them both together after each isolated stroking.

It may take a while to build a connection like more than one or two sessions or it could be almost immediately. If you practice enough you will build a connection, so keep doing it. Connect your clitoris to all the other sensitive areas of your genitals such as the introitus and the other labia. Once you build a connection it will make intercourse a great deal more pleasurable.

Involving the Clitoris Directly

Another possibility is stroking the clitoris with either your own hand or with the guy's hand while engaged in coitus. This makes intercourse a little more work but again can be productive in producing female orgasm. If the woman has another area such as her nipples that are connected already to her clitoris then she or he can stimulate those while doing the act.

The other possibility for getting the clitoris more involved is by experimenting with different positions while having intercourse. Some women have reported benefits from being on top and riding forward on the male penis. You can also experiment with pillows to get a better angle to involve clitoral stimulation with either the male or female on top. If the woman has a responsive area of her vagina like the G-spot, it is possible by getting in a position that stimulates this area that she can also have an orgasmic reaction.

We think that the most important of all these methods is making sure that the female genitals are engorged and aroused before starting, just like the male has to be that way before he can begin any kind of penetration with his penis.

A woman is usually the one who decides whether they the couple will have intercourse. Some women do it even though they don't enjoy it because they think that they should or that it is their duty. I think that a lot of women have had intercourse when they would have preferred to be stimulated in another way. I also believe that the more a woman learns about how her body works and the pivotal importance of her clitoris that her desire for other than coital intimacy will only increase. That is why it is so important for both the man and the woman to learn how to arouse her properly. Never have intercourse if it does not feel good, especially if it hurts. We had a couple of friends who would have intercourse with their husbands because they thought they should even though it was not fun. They often would get urinary tract infections afterwards.

Sex and sensuality are one of the most if not the most fun activity that people can have and really is an art that has to be learned. Any person or animal can have intercourse but to have a great orgasm requires a lot more skill and training.

Orgasm and Health

Scientific research indicates that orgasm has health benefits such as boosting the immune system and improving a woman's bladder control, but I know of no research specifically focused on the relaxed extended orgasms that we explore and write about. By improving sleep and reducing stress, sexual activity also contributes to your overall appearance.

Look and Feel Younger

In one study, British psychologist Dr. David Weeks reported that men and women looked seven years younger when they had intercourse more often than the ones who looked older. It was based on people's responses to a quiz that he handed out over ten years. You could slip that around, of course, and make the case they having more sex because they looked better than others their age.

In a Welsh study in 1997, it was found that men had a lower risk of cardiovascular disease if they had more frequent sex. Again, you could turn it around and speculate they were having more sex because they had better cardiovascular systems.

In a study done in 2000 by Carol Ellison and reported by Beverly Whipple in her book *The Orgasm Answer Guide*, it was shown that the hormone oxytocin is increased into the bloodstream from the hypothalamus during orgasm. Oxytocin is good for relieving stress and is known as the "love" hormone as it creates a feeling of closeness to one's partner. It is also released during other bonding activities such as a parent cuddling a child, or good friends having a heart-to-heart chat.

Dr. Whipple also reported in studying women who masturbated regularly that their pain tolerance increased. Endorphins are released with orgasm so people should feel better.

Using MRI, Barry Komisaruk and Nan Wise measured blood flow in the brains of a number of women who were masturbating. They found an increase in blood flow to all parts of their brains. If you want to jump to a conclusion, you might use this to argue that orgasm helps women to think clearly!

PMS

We have seen numerous clients who had bad cramps and head-aches during their menses; we recommended having more frequent and better orgasms as a possible cure. Orgasm will increase the blood flow to the uterine area and the contractions from the orgasm will quicken the removal of the menstrual blood that is possibly causing the cramps. And the endorphins and dopamine hormones released with orgasm relieve pain. We suggest to our students that to avoid or lessen their PMS to have at least daily orgasms starting four or five days before expecting their period and continuing this routine into the first couple days of bleeding or longer.

Having good and frequent orgasms is also beneficial to women who are going through menopause. Vera and a number of other women who had a healthy sex life with lots of EMOs had an easier transition than the average woman.

More Benefits of Orgasm

I don't know if having a regular diet of orgasm will make you live longer but I definitely think you will have a more joyous life. I am sure there are lots of old people out there whose sex lives were not all that great and many people who died prematurely who had a good sex life. There are just too many other factors and variables that would make it difficult to prove either way.

I know for myself that everything appears more positive or better after getting off. Food tastes better. My face looks more relaxed. All my senses including creativity seem to improve. I like my life situation more. My mood is enhanced, at least for a time. If it is late at night, we even sleep better. Extended orgasm increases our circulation.

There is probably a difference if you have an orgasm in a relaxed state versus a tensed up one to what your body feels like afterwards. I know some women who reported that they feel different after the two different ways. When they have a relaxed body orgasm, they continue to feel their pussy afterwards. They are more alert and more turned on. When they tense up and go over the so-called edge, their turn-on and general aliveness is not as keen. In either case, they report to be more joyous.

I also think that people are nicer after getting off. This is my opinion. They are less stingy with their attention and affection and not as needy as someone who has not experienced this pleasure. This can be due to the increased oxytocin levels or of PEA (Phenyl Ethyl Amine) another "love hormone" that supposedly is increased after orgasm and when a person falls in love. It is also found in small amounts in chocolate. One has to eat a lot of chocolate to get enough PEA and the side effects such as weight gain from eating a lot of chocolate are not as kind as compared to those of an orgasm.

We also believe that most people and especially women who experience relaxed and extended orgasms will make better decisions after getting off. This is probably because they are in a better mental state, less anxious and can see the big picture with more clarity. We have noticed that women who have trained to have EMOs are financially healthier than before they learned about their orgasmic potential. We collected no statistically valid data on these claims, but it makes sense that someone who is more gratified and joyous with her life situation will attract, create and notice more of the positive manifestations than someone who is less gratified.

What is the "appropriate" amount of orgasm to produce the optimum health and to feel the best? What is the proper extent of orgasm to being the most joyous and grateful? Is *more* always better or does it depend on the individual? Is there a point where it becomes unhealthy? These are all valid questions, but I do not believe there are any valid answers to them yet. Quality of the orgasm is undoubtedly more important than quantity. But if the quality is there, what would the correct quantity be for peak well-being? Is one great one better than three really good ones?

Negative Effects

I did an online search on the negative effects of orgasm. According to William Last in an Internet article, there are some negative consequences to having orgasm—at least if you're a rat. He claims that after orgasmic sex, male's androgen receptors decrease and this lack of testosterone binding sites causes males to feel stressful and anxious as well as tired after having an orgasm. Their dopamine levels fall too. Females have a similar but more delayed response. This study is only in regard to coital orgasms. These rats have not taken our courses and learned how to do each other manually. Additionally, they have not learned how to be relaxed when receiving one.

According to this article, the male rat's view of his partner is not as enthusiastically pro as it was before having sex. With the introduction of a new receptive partner, he regains his edge as his dopamine levels rise again.

We believe that the art of learning how to be relaxed for humans and how to manually stimulate your partner to that perfect place of gratification without overdoing it will keep them gratified yet hungry for more and not jeopardize one's emotional state.

William Last then brings up the "Coolidge Effect," which is a fairly well known but a cute story. President Coolidge and his wife were touring a chicken farm. The farmer proclaimed how his rooster goes all day long, day after day, copulating with the chickens. The First Lady liked that idea and asked the farmer to relate that to the President. When the farmer told Calvin C. this anecdote, Coolidge asked, "Does he do this with the same hen?" "No, replied the farmer." "Please tell that to Mrs. Coolidge." said the President. Supposedly female rats are also more receptive when a new male is thrown into the cage with her.

I did notice when I was living in a commune of over one hundred people that when a new guy showed up many of the females who were living there already, perked up. A lot of the females would check this new male out sexually. After a month or so of thinking he was in heaven things would go back to normal. He was no longer being pursued and his sex life would dry up fast unless one of the women decided to keep him as a partner. Of course, it was similar when a new female joined the group, as the males would want to check her out, too. This activity was more dependent on her turn-on as to how long this attention would continue and from whom.

There are meeting places for so called sexual addicts to go to, to do the twelve steps just as with Alcoholics Anonymous. Supposedly according to William Last these sexual addicts are trying to amp up their dopamine levels. I think most of these folks are probably psychologically unhealthy. I don't think that the orgasm is the root problem, however, if they are like that rooster then they are probably not functioning very well in relationships. Also, I would tend to believe that the problem for most of these addicts is too much fucking and not too much doing by manual stimulation.

We had some courses where most of the women who were living at the commune were required to have many relaxed orgasms daily. Everyone seemed to benefit from this attention including the males who were with these women. The orgasms were mandatory and if not completed by a certain weekly period the person would face some kind of "punishment" or a fine. Nobody complained and there were only a few "lawbreakers." After the course was over the quantity of orgasms drastically declined. The fun level went down, but no one seemed abnormally dysfunctional because of it. This seemed to prove none of these women had become addicted to orgasm.

We have found no problems for women getting extended orgasms as long as you use proper lubrication.

Choosing to have an orgasmic existence and learning your sexual potential is a wonderful asset in having a great life situation. The positives far outweigh the negatives and the chance of becoming an addict is minimal if you are psychologically healthy to begin with.

3
Self-Pleasuring

Whether you are with a partner or by yourself, it is always your responsibility to promote your own pleasure. This chapter is dedicated to self-pleasuring, or masturbation. Masturbation is a path to the divine gift of sexual pleasure, and it can be fine-tuned through certain practices to realize one's true sensual beingness. This practice is to learn to stay present with your sensations, to be with your pleasure.

One of the tricks in being pleasured is to pretend that it is happening to you. To be at effect where you can surrender to pleasure. When you are with a partner it is easier to pretend that you are not at cause; that you are the pleasure victim of something outside of you. The reality is that you are always at cause but when you are with someone else it is easier to forget that you created everything. This chapter will give you some ideas on how to become your own pleasure victim.

Being that we love to talk about sex, Vera and I will often ask our friends and our students, too, how their sex lives are. We get a mixture of responses. Nobody says that it is none of your business because they know what our business is. Sometimes they will complain and say that they have no one to make out with. We then will ask them how about self-pleasuring? Some of them will report that they are having a great time doing it and others will grumble some more about not wanting to do that or how it is better with a partner.

I have news for them and for you, perhaps. You can have more fun pleasuring yourself than you ever dreamed of. I know that from experience. I cherish the moments I spend with me. It is an opportunity to not only have a great time but to explore and learn and be creative. I think that even if one has an amazing partner as I do, it is not an excuse to become lazy and have them always do it for you or to you. Spend some alone time and learn and then appreciate how well you know yourself and how well you can create pleasure for yourself. It is a chance to have immense fun and to pleasurably discover more about you. There is always something new to learn and to explore about your body and its relationship to pleasure.

In our previous books we laid out an extensive list of exercises in precise order to access further knowledge of your body to do on your own. Briefly, there are six of them.

- Visiting Dignity—Set up your space, make it look nice and gather something for each of your senses, like music, food, fragrant flowers, and so on.
- Mirror Exercise—Look at your naked body with appreciation not negative judging.
- Tactile Inventory—Touch yourself anywhere on your body except genitals for the pleasure of it.
- Focal Point Exercise—Choose a focal point like your inner elbow and touch around it pleasurably in circular fashion to create tension, where it wants to be touched also.
- Masturbation for Pleasurable Effect—Pleasure your genitals by stroking them but not going over the edge.
- Connections—Connect different body parts to your clitoris or penis by stroking them at the same time.

They are extremely helpful and if you have never done them, then it would behoove you to get our EMO books and practice them. If you did them all properly it would take a good couple of hours or longer. It is not something that you do only once but best to do them regularly and continually over your lifespan. The Visiting Dignitary and the Mirror exercise may be the most important ones.

Here I am taking some of the training wheels off and giving you freer rein or latitude to do whatever feels good to you in regard to self-pleasuring. We are giving you some easier or less demanding options that may have been covered in previous books. If you like music, have some music in the background. If you do not care for music, then don't. If you like to eat or drink something when taking a break from stimulating your body, then have some close by. If you don't care, just skip it. Each time is a new experience, and you don't have to do the same thing every time.

Time Victims

Some people protest that exercises we recommend to get to know yourself take too much time. Well we are taking that excuse away. Doing the exercises in the proper sequence given has numerous benefits, such as: tumescing your body to where it feels more, expanding your awareness to include loving your body more, and in creating the best space to feel the most. That being said, not everyone has that much time available to do the whole set, each time. It is better to do some or part of the exercises than none at all.

Take whatever time you want, whether it is one minute or an hour or more. Just because you do it longer does not make it better. Quality is far more important than quantity.

If you feel like exploring your body in the mirror go ahead and explore and if you don't feel like doing that, that is fine also. If you want to do a quick observation, instead of your whole body, then do that. Maybe do one new angle or one new viewpoint that you had not thought of before. If you want to go straight to your genitals and skip all the preliminary touching exercises that is okay too. If you just want to do the focal point exercise or just want to do the mirror exercise then do those. It is your body and please do what you feel like doing each time. Use the options you have as just that, options. Always choose for what will be the most pleasurable selections and don't feel guilty for your choices later. It is also okay to feel a little challenged or discomfort with selecting something new or different than usual in order to expand your horizons. Pleasure can come in different forms. You can always stop whenever you have had enough.

Focal Point Exercise

There are a few exercises that it seems most people either don't do at all or do only once or twice. One of the original exercises that we wrote about and people tend to forget was creating focal points on different areas of your body. A focal point is any spot you choose, and by deliberately not touching it but stroking lightly the area around it in circles. For that reason I wanted to write a full description here This is an exercise of tumescing a spot on your body and is useful when you are playing with your partner too; for example, when you get closer and closer to her clitoris.

Playing around with different focal points can be helpful to get you in a sensual mood without jumping straight to your genitals. It can be used in conjunction with the tactile exercise where you are exploring different areas of your body with what kind of touches feel best. I know that I would often only do the tactile exercise and skip the focal point one before doing the genital self-pleasuring.

Because I knew I was writing a new description of self-pleasuring, I played with the focal point exercise. I found it quite stimulating. I explored some areas that I was discussing in the pleasuring a woman section such as using my knuckles and the areas in between my fingers that can be called the webbing. I wanted to see if I could create more sensation in my own hands. Those areas are quite sensitive to touch. Those areas plus my fingers themselves and the palm of my hand were all easily aroused to pleasure. I did this specific hand focal point exercises a couple of times. I cannot say for sure that I created increased sensitivity (time will tell) but I was surprised how sensitive these areas are. I also played around without using my fingertips at all. I created focal points with my knuckles on knuckles and knuckles on palm and on webbing. Then I tried palm on palm. It really felt like someone else was touching me when I did not use my fingertips. This is one simple example of how to fool yourself into being at effect and becoming your own pleasure beneficiary.

For clarification, in this next description you may use your fingertips. Just pick out one specific spot such as the middle of your palm to be your focal point and see what happens when you gently touch close to it but not directly on it. It starts to crave your touch. By circling around it but never quite getting there, you will be continually stoking this desire. To finish or complete the particular focal point you can finally touch it firmly and deliberately, remaining on the area until the tumescence is alleviated. By putting more attention on your hands by doing these exercises it will be beneficial to you when pleasuring your partner with them. Combining this exercise with the connections exercise to be described shortly will probably be the most advantageous combination. Your hands and fingers will become more sensitive.

The focal point exercises are also fun and may get you into the mood for having a more enjoyable orgasm while self-pleasuring. It is also something that you can add on to tumesce your partner before you get to their genitals. You can also create a focal spot of the clitoris or the area under the head of the penis. When I am doing a woman the clitoris is always a quasi-focal point even though I am touching elsewhere. I always have at least some attention on it.

Take however much time, or as little, as you want to do the focal point exercise and any others. Just because you do it longer does not make it better; quality is far more important than quantity.

MEO

I like to joke that you can't give yourself an EMO but you can give yourself a MEO. This can be an acronym for Massive Extended Orgasm or Masturbatory Extended Orgasm.

Pre-Lubrication Masturbation

You do not have to stimulate your genitals every time that you are self-pleasuring but more than likely most times you will want to. We have known some women who could have orgasms by touching themselves in areas that they had previously connected to their clitorises. Some women can have an orgasm just by putting attention on their genitals or by fantasizing on erotica. Try just lying there and putting your attention on your genitals.

Sometimes I will start with light strokes through my clothes if I am not already naked to get a little more in the mood (without lubricant of course). Once you remove your clothes you don't have to start immediately with lubricant though I sometimes do. I like to wrap my hand around my penis, which is often quite hot, with my hand that is often quite cold, and feel the sensation built first without lubricant and then maybe with. At other times I will just put a finger on it without moving and notice how it feels. Each time out is an opportunity to be creative and curious about how your body works and how it responds to different stimuli.

If you have a pussy instead of a penis we also suggest exploring diverse touches all over your genitals. Check out your perineum, your labia, your vaginal opening, on top of your hood, from below your clitoris and along the sides of your clitoral hood. Try pressing gently, changing the pressure, poking, tugging, spreading, pulling or whatever feels good to do.

Exposing the Clitoris

It would be a good idea to become proficient at properly pulling back on the hood to expose the clitoris. Practice exposing your clitoris from under the hood without touching it directly so you can learn how to do that easily. You can bend over to get a good visual of how your hood is attached and how much pressure you need to pull it back and expose the clitoris. You can use your hand mirror placed properly in order to aid you to see what you are doing.

You can first try to pull it back with both hands and then refine it to just one hand, so that you will have a free hand available to eventually stroke the clitoris. Place your hands just above the hood and clitoris on the Mons Pubis and pull upward and press against it at the same time. You want to use enough pressure to expose the clitoris but not too much so that the pleasure becomes affected. You can use your fingertips or your palms, or any part of your hand. You may have to experiment for the best way to do this. You can also try pressing against the side of the hood and pushing it upward away from the clitoris, with a finger or your thumb. Once the clitoris is stimulated and becomes fully engorged, it will pop out of the hood and you won't have to continually pull on the hood.

Remember, like snowflakes, everybody's genitals are different. Women's clitorises come in all shapes and sizes. Some have a tight hood and others have a hood that retracts easily. Some have a hood that will not retract at all, while others may have hardly a hood at all. Labia too came in many forms and can be large or tiny.

Vibrators

We highly recommend using your hands to masturbate, as opposed to using a vibrator or humping something like a pillow. We have had many female students that have used a vibrator extensively, previous to studying with us. For many of these women, stimulating their genitals with a vibrator was the only way that they could reach an orgasm. The problem with vibrators is just that. The person using them becomes dependent on them and they can no longer have an orgasm with their partner or by their own hand.

We are not totally against vibrators. There are many different types of vibrators, and I would be the first to admit to not being an expert on them. Perhaps there are some that are better than others. I know that the sexologist, Betty Dodson, wrote a whole book dedicated to them, called *Sex for One*.

However, from what we have seen, most vibrators tend to numb the orgasmic response when women want to learn to be pleasured by hand or mouth or even with intercourse. For that reason, we have women who wish to study with us give up their vibrators while they are taking our course. The body learns to feel more again without having that constant electric stimulation. They can always use their toys, once they are finished with our class.

Once you learn to have great orgasms with your own hand, then you can decide when and if you still want to use your vibrator.

Pleasurable Lubrication For Women

For women, the application of lubricant is about pleasure and curiosity. You can save the head of your clitoris for last and begin applying the lubricant on your perineum, anus (if washed beforehand), introitus, or your inner labia to waken up those areas to pleasure. Check out as many different kinds of pleasurable lubricating strokes that you can think of on the different areas of your labia or anywhere on your lubricated genitals in any order that you please.

The strokes can vary with pressure, how many fingers to use, the speed of the stroke as well as the location. You can apply the lubricant to all areas quickly or take your time spreading it to the different areas. You then can stroke the chosen areas after lubricating them in any way that you like in order to determine what feels best and to tumesce yourself where your clitoris wants to be included in the fun.

Here are some ideas: You can press a small single spot on the perineum, the inner labia, the anus, or on the introitus, repeatedly or just briefly. You can stroke a larger area, up and down or round and round. You can stroke the lubricant on gently in a small region or on a wider area.

A lot of women are very sensitive on the top of their labia that are close to their clitoris. Many of our students like a quick up and down stroke with very gentle pressure on the upper part of their labia or all the way up and down the labia, once it has been lubricated. You can do the two labia separately or at the same time, using two fingers or two hands. Check out how it feels to get closer and closer to the bottom of your clitoris until you finally bump up against it with your fingertip.

Don't lubricate your pubic hair. If you shave then it would be okay to lubricate those areas too. It is not necessary to lubricate your outer labia, and do not lubricate your hood, as it will make it slippery and difficult to pull it back later, when you wish to stroke your clitoris. If it does get lubricated, you can always wipe it off with your small towel (We like to use a small dry washcloth).

Some women and some men may enjoy lightly putting a little bit of lubricant on their nipples and then stroking them lightly or with whatever pressure feels best. Notice any responses in your genitals at the same time. See how your nipples can control your genitals. You may be a pleasure victim again. I enjoy starting with my facial lips and putting a little lubricant there. I have a connection and I can feel sensation starting to build in my penis at the same time.

Feel free to create and use any spreading of lubricant ideas that you come up with.

Pleasurable Self-Stroking a Clitoris

There are so many variations of touches and areas to lubricate and to play with that you could not possibly do them all in one session. Do as much of the above ideas as you enjoy, create new ideas and remember which ones you liked the best. Next time you can try out different ideas. It is a good idea to create a Sensual Journal with some of your ideas and accomplishments.

If you tumesced yourself well, now is the time to check out the head of your clitoris.

You can go directly with your lubricated fingertip and apply it to the head of your clitoris or you can continue teasing yourself by holding your finger almost on it and just feel your own attention.

Once you are ready to lubricate and touch the head of the clitoris you will have to get your hood pulled back to expose the clitoral head. Pull back your hood as you have previously practiced, and apply some lubricant to the tip of your index or middle finger and coat your clitoral head. Depending on the size of the clitoris you can coat it all at once or one quadrant at a time.

Now that you have applied the lubricant you can put the lubricant aside. With the water-soluble type you will either keep it close by for reapplying it or keep a little cup of water handy to reconstitute it when it becomes too sticky.

It is probably better to start with a light touch and then check out different pressures to find the exact force that feels best. Check the different quadrants of your clitoris especially the upper left to see if that area is the most sensitive as it is in the majority of women.

Try stroking the clitoris in a rhythmical pattern on the same area for as many strokes in a row that you can feel enjoyably. We think the tip of the finger in a small area usually is best. As soon as you notice that you are no longer feeling as much as you were on the previous stroke, take a break.

You can use small strokes in one little area or quadrant. Some women when first exploring their clitoris find it too sensational to stay directly on the clitoris for many strokes in a row and prefer longer strokes that go on and off their clitoris. It is best to use a rhythmical repeated stroke and then when you want to change the stroke to a different type to again use this new repeated pattern.

You can try different pressures, different speeds, different locations as well as different lengths. You can try the up and down stroke as well as little or larger circular ones. This is your time to experiment. Be creative. These are just some ideas that you can employ if you like. Once you have been stroking yourself for a certain length of time your clitoris will probably become more and more engorged. It also will become easier to touch, as it will engorge away from its hood that was covering it.

Super Sensitive Clitoris

Some women are super sensitive and have a fear of touching their clitoris directly, by themselves, and even more fearful with a partner. We have found that in almost all these cases, a slow and deliberate approach will overcome this fearful sensitivity.

Experiment on finding out the limits, where it changes from pleasure to trepidation. This can mean touching the clitoris through the hood or perhaps just touching nearby, either below or above it. Check out if it feels good to apply some lubricant on your clitoris without stroking it. You can try using a larger amount of lubricant, where your finger can rub the lubricant but not be touching the skin of the clitoris directly. Instead of stroking your clitoris, you can press your finger against the clitoris and then releasing it. If that is okay then you can press again and so on. Don't start stroking until you feel righteous about doing so. When you do start stroking directly use very light pressure and only do a few strokes at a time. If you take your time and proceed slowly I promise that you will eventually learn to appreciate the direct touches right on it.

Any progress that you make is going in a positive direction. It may take more than one or two sessions to overcome your fear although we have had some students that were originally fearful, who got to the point of direct stimulation on their first session. Remember to stay in the moment, quiet your mind so that you are not thinking and comparing yourself to anyone else or any preconceived preferences. The goal is to have pleasure with each stroke and not to have any specific expectations.

Two Hands for Women

Once your clitoris is fully engorged and is easier to touch; you can use your second hand to do other enjoyable additional maneuvers. These exercises can be many fold. Some examples are playing with your labia, your perineum or your introitus or even your nipple at the same time as you are stroking your clitoris. Play with as small or as large an area as you want.

You can insert one or more fingers inside your vagina as you are simultaneously stroking your clitoris. Only use insertion if it feels pleasurable to do. You can place and direct your fingers up or down or to the side. There are a number of areas inside the vagina that many women seem to enjoy. Stroke with as much pressure and as deeply as it feels best. The upper side of the vagina includes the G-Spot area which is at the top anterior area of the vagina kind of right under where the clitoris is or a couple of inches or so deep. Use a come hither type of stroke to stimulate it. The clitoris has a shaft and roots in addition to its external head. The G-Spot area is in the area where the nerve roots of the clitoris are located and one of the reasons that it feels so pleasurable to some women to be touched there.

The clitoral shaft can also be fun for some women to play with. It will engorge at the same time that your clitoral head is engorged. You can stroke it at the same time you stroke the head of your clitoris or squeeze it between your finger and thumb. If your clitoral head is too sensitive to be touched directly you can try stroking the shaft instead.

You can also play with your anus as it has the second highest concentration of nerve endings after the clitoris. Use enough lubricant and start with gentle touches. You can always add more pressure and insertion if you like.

Pleasurable Lubrication For Men

Sometimes all I will do is apply the lubricant sensually to myself, which could take a few minutes and then wiping it off with a towel. It can be that much fun. It is sheer joy. I will work my way from one area of the penis to another, slowly but surely, like starting from the dorsal or less sensitive side, then the lower ventral side, to finally getting onto the apex. You can also take your time with the lubricant application and then continue with more stroking.

Other times I will put a glob of lubricant on my middle and index fingers and spread it quickly all over the penis, almost at once. Once it is coated you can hold it gently but firmly with your whole hand. You can feel the heat, possible throbbing, and engorgement occurring. Take a deep breath and relax into the sensation. Make sure that your hand feels pleasured, as well as your penis. You can apply some pressure, starting from a little and then increasing the pressure, as long as it still feels good to do so, until you determine what is enough, and what feels best.

You have a choice of how many fingers to use to apply the lubricant. If you are trying the slow method then one finger is probably best. Sometimes I will even put a little gob of the stuff on one area at a time with one finger without spreading it around till my whole penis has these little gobs of lubricant all over it. Then I will spread it slowly, still with one finger, till the whole penis is coated completely.

At other times I will take a larger gob of lubricant on all my fingers at once and circle my penis with that hand and quickly or even slowly if I so desire, coat the penis so that there are no dry spots left. That means I may just hold my hand there or move it just slightly and deliberately up and down my shaft or around and around it and feel the cool lubricant against my flesh. My attention is on wherever my hand is and I am enjoying the sensation to its fullest.

You can use fingertips to spread the lubricant or use the part of the fingers further toward the palm. Another way to spread the lubricant is by keeping your fingers straight, not circling the whole penis at once and gently applying the lubricant on the penis with either a back and forth motion or a more circular movement. It is your time to be creative and to experiment with as many ways as you can think of. By being playful here you are learning to touch yourself just for the fun of it and not to necessarily get anywhere in specific.

The most important factor in applying the lubricant and in the whole masturbatory experience is to enjoy what you are doing and to feel with as much of your attention that you can at all times. If you find yourself not feeling much and that your mind is wandering take a short break and then put your attention back where it does you the most good. Maybe move to a different area on your genitals. Just putting on the lubricant can be a fantastic personal party and we want you to enjoy this self-celebration to its fullest extent. The lubricant is an external tool so you can pretend that it is putting you at effect and that you are becoming a pleasure victim to the lubricant. "The lubricant made me do it."

Though I might tease myself by not putting on the lubricant on my most sensitive penis area till last (creating a lubrication focal point), I will eventually cover the entire penis with lubricant before beginning any serious stroking.

Smearing it on the pubic hair can be messy and is unwarranted. I don't usually put any on my scrotum but you can play around and experiment there too if you like. If your anus is clean, then you play with that by applying lubricant and first gently stroking and experiment with different pressures.

Some Ideas for Self-Pleasuring a Penis

You can take one hand and wrap it around your penis touching as much surface area as you can. You can check out squeezing it to find out your favorite pressure. You can check out this whole hand technique while moving it up and down keeping the hand from twisting, again to determine the best pressure and your favorite speed. You can then check out how it feels to move your hand in a circular motion clockwise and counter clockwise around your penis without moving it up and down. Go in one direction as far as you can without having it hurt your hand. You can play with twisting your hand in a helical motion around your penis as you go up and down or just twisting in one small location. It will depend also on how big your penis and your hand are. You can move your penis around as you hold it in your hand as if playing with a gearshift. You can hold it in your hand and pull and tug on it using different pressures.

Whatever stroke you are using It is usually a good idea to duplicate the identical strokes rhythmically and repeatedly to take the pleasure higher and create more intensity. We don't want you to squirt too soon so back off or stop when you feel that you are getting close. Then you can change to a different stroke or go back to the same one.

Another stroke you can check out is using a single fingertip or a couple of fingers along the sensitive side of your penis. You can also do a similar stroke with your thumb. Find what spots and areas are most sensitive and enjoyable to touch. You can go all the way up and down your entire penis or do a similar stroke in just a small area. Again you can vary the pressure and speed to determine what you enjoy the most.

A lot of guys do it hard and fast and we would like you to put some intention on doing it more gently and slower. Once you get close to ejaculating and have taken a break and started again, if you have not stopped for a long period, it probably won't take long to get back up to that point again. This edge is a place where you can create a lot of amazing pleasure as you experiment with your body. It may be that only a couple of strokes bring you back to the edge, so be aware and prescient.

Second-Hand for Men

You can use your second hand to perform a number of possible activities. You can if you are engorged, stroke your penis with both hands so that you have even more contact. You can go up and down together staying on the penis the whole time with both hands. You may take one hand at a time up your shaft and over the head of your penis and then removing it. At the same time that you are removing one hand start with the other hand down below at the base of the penis and bring that up. Continuously repeat one hand after the other, changing the speed or the pressure or the timing. This way there is always one hand on the penis at least. The stroking is always in the up direction to create a rhythmical pattern. One can also check out only going in the downward direction. If you have a really engorged large sized penis or small hands you can do a two handed stroke in both directions leaving the hands on the penis at all times. Another way to do that would be to make a ring out of your index finger and thumb circled around your penis and use one or both hands to slide up and down the shaft.

You can also add on your second hand to play with your testicles or under your testicles where you can feel your hidden cock aka internal extension of your penis that probably has some engorgement. Right under the testicles on the perineum if you press deep enough through the hidden cock you can put some pressure on your prostate area. You can control your ejaculation by pressing here with just the right pressure. You can also stimulate this area to increase sensation with a lighter touch.

Keep stroking your penis as you were doing before with whatever stroke you are using. If you are pressing your prostate area to stop from ejaculating it is a good idea to stop stroking your penis until the urge goes away. Touch these secondary areas with different kinds of strokes too and different pressures. Being that I like women's legs I have even used my own by bending it so that I can get my foot under my testicles. This is another example of putting oneself at effect and pretending someone else is doing it to you.

It is pleasurable to most guys to pull on their testicles rather than to push them into the body. Try it without lubricant and then with. Use both hands at the same time. The anus has a lot of nerve receptors and can be enjoyable to stroke. Start gently and definitely use lubricant, as it is erectile tissue. Some people like more pressure and even insertion and prostate massage. Proceed slowly and incrementally if this is something that you have never done before. Some men like to massage their prostate from inside their anus. Some other ideas on using your second hand will be presented in the *Connections* section that follows.

For both genders, once you become experienced at self-pleasuring you will know your favorite ways to be touched. Your peaks will become longer and women will be able to directly touch their clitoral head. We suggest that you keep an open mind and continue looking for new creative ways to pleasure you. Pleasure can be found in numerous adaptations so even though you have found specific touches that you like best you may find some new ones to add on to your repertoire. So be creative.

Connections

Connections exercises are vitally beneficial, so try to add them onto your important list of sensual research. If you can build some connections your body will be that much more orgasmic and pleasure conscious.

Once the primary or main genital area or, specifically, the clitoris of a woman and the penis of a man is in high sensation feeling mode then you can start with building the connection. All you have to do is to start stroking a secondary area at the same time that you are stroking your primary one with basically a similar kind of stroke; speed wise and pressure wise and even length wise. This secondary area can be your facial lip, your genital labia, your nipple, and your introitus, which is the vaginal opening of a woman, or even your anus or any body part you would like to connect. We recommend that you use lubricant on any area that you will be stroking for an extended time, especially erectile tissue.

When you have both the primary and secondary areas feeling pleasure at the same time, you take your hand off of the secondary area. You may leave your hand right above your skin and even continue with the motion as if you were touching it. Notice if there is any sensation in that area that you have stopped touching. If there is no sensation, put your hand back on and continue stroking both areas in synch. When you first do this exercise, you may not notice any sensation so don't feel that it is not working. Keep practicing.

After you have been stroking both areas again to a nice responsiveness, take your hand off of your primary area. Leave your hand right above your genitals and again continue with the motion an inch or less above it. Again, notice if you have any sensation in your penis or clitoris as you continue to pleasurably stroke your secondary area. If there is no sensation, then put your hand back on your genitals and continue to stroke both areas at the same time with the same motion.

Keep doing this, that is, stroking both areas in synch and then removing your hand off of one, together and then one area only, together and then the other area. Notice any response when you remove your hand. Keep your hand off until the sensation goes away if you indeed feel something. Then begin stroking them in synch together again after the sensation fades away. It may take some time, that is numerous sessions before you get any concrete results but even a tingle or some warmth is a good sign. Once you get one area connected the next area will be that much easier to add on. Once you build a connection by continuing to practice, it will get stronger and stronger. You may become a pleasure victim of your own lips.

I am just over seventy now and took my first class in sensuality over forty-five years ago. I did my homework and eventually built a strong connection between my facial lips (both the upper and lower) and my penis. Often, since I built a connection, I will begin a masturbation or self-pleasuring session by putting a little lubricant on my lips and touching them sensually. I will touch either my upper or lower one or both depending on what feels right at the time. The lubricant and touch feels great directly on them and the connection spreads to my genitals and penis so I start feeling down there before touching them. I can play with my lips for however long I feel like it from a few seconds to a number of minutes. I can touch myself with whatever pressure or speed feels the most pleasurable at that moment and this can vary from session to session and even the phases in one stint. Then after putting some lubricant on my penis and doing some stroking on an already turned-on area I can add my lips back into the fray and use one hand stroking on my penis and the other hand stroking my lips. The combination is awesome and since I often pleasure myself where I am peaking close to the edge without going over, I can take my hand off the close to squirting penis and keep it at the edge with the lip stroking continuing.

I have also found a strong connection above my penis around the area of my lower abdomen. After I am feeling it in my genitals and the sensations are in a steadily increasing mode, I will add some pressure to my lower abdomen at the same time or in place of the direct stroking on my penis and this will also take me higher without spilling too much ejaculate at once. The trick is that I had to first do my connections exercises diligently in order that these areas became available to use as an additional boost while self-pleasuring.

Connecting Throat and Sounds

If you are quiet by nature or shy when making love it might do you some good to make some noise when being pleasured even when you are all by yourself. It is not to make sound just for the sake of making sound but to feel the orgasm in your throat area and harness the deep guttural sounds that reflect how you are feeling. If you live with other people such as your family and kids and you don't want them to know what you are doing you always have the option of doing yourself quietly. If you do get a chance where you are alone in your home or hotel room, check out connecting your voice to your genitals.

It does not have to be extremely loud but enough so that you can feel the pleasure of doing it.

I seem to use this technique when I am at some high point or peak of arousal; it's not something I do constantly during the extended orgasm. When I do connect my throat to the sensation of the orgasm emanating from my genitals it adds to the total experience and can even extend that peak as well as increase the sensation. As with the connection to my lips and abdomen I can just make the sounds when I am at an intense point to keep the orgasm going without stroking directly on my penis.

I have included a section in the communication chapter that expands on the ideas in the last couple of paragraphs. I will relate some of the specific sounds one can use to connect your throat to your genitals and even how to connect real words.

Pornography and Fantasy

We are of the opinion that as long as you are not totally obsessed with your fantasies or with using pornography that they can be helpful aids while self-pleasuring. I have used both though not usually at the same time while masturbating although porn really is fantasy too. I think that men in general like using pornography a lot more than women do. I sometimes will use pornography, as a means to start feeling more turned-on in the beginning of a self-pleasuring session and then close my eyes and get in a more comfortable position. I then may use the fantasy version of what I just watched or another fantasy entirely to continue with my pleasuring. Fantasy is probably used by both sexes equally, but the fantasy material is different. It is not mandatory to use fantasy, but it is another way to become at effect of yourself and feel like someone other than you is doing it to you. Fantasy is free and the only barrier is your imagination.

We will go into some deeper specific fantasy material and how to play with your own and your partner's imagination in the communication chapter.

4

Overcoming Resistances

Recently we received an interesting business proposal. The proposal was to put a course on the Internet describing a "Do-Date." The fellow who proposed this endeavor said most people don't know what a Do-Date is so you will have to start from scratch. The expression is not my favorite because it kind of sounds like when a woman is slated to give birth or when your library book is due. For that reason, I have not used that expression myself very often but have used the similar expressions: "Would you like to get done?" or "Can I do you?" or even "Will you do me?" I have also regularly used the term "doing someone." At this point I have not decided whether to do the Internet thing about "Doing" or "Do Date" but thought I would include it here since it is a good idea whether in print or otherwise.

Doing someone used to have the connotation of intercourse. This all changed for some of us in the late 1960s and early 1970s when Dr. Vic Baranco created the Basic Sensuality Course and used the phrase to infer that you were offering someone an orgasmic possibility by stroking them on the genitals with your hands. It could be the pleasuring of a clitoris or a penis but no longer assumed that there would be any penis into vagina penetration.

People have been stimulating each other with hands for probably as long as they have had hands. Doing a guy or rubbing on a penis to pleasure him has been happening for millennia by the so-called "oldest profession" or prostitution. Of course, prostitution has not been mainstreamed in most societies. However, every society has had some version of females selling their sexual favors. The better one is at most any profession the more repeat customers, which is good for business. Therefore, it was and still is necessary to learn one's craft. Besides learning from experience, these sexual sellers often learned techniques and skills from their more experienced sisters.

The pleasuring of a clitoris or the doing of a woman with hands although it is as long-standing probably as the doing of a penis has not been studied or taught in any reported fashion in probably all of history until recently. Most men throughout antiquity probably had very little information about actually pleasuring a woman to orgasm. Perhaps there were a few societies where there was a more liberal attitude toward pleasure such as the Karma Sutra times in ancient India or some isolated Pacific Islanders. I have not heard of any in the way of manually stimulating a woman's clitoris.

Although the head of the clitoris has more nerve endings than the penis; men have been able to have an easier time with having an orgasm than women. This is because of this lack of knowledge as well as the fact that the clitoris is more hidden. The pleasuring of a woman or specifically giving her orgasmic gratification by stimulating her clitoris with one's hands has become our life's work. So, yes, is the answer to the question does orgasm matter? It matters for a woman as much as it matters to a man. It is simply one of life's biggest bonuses and to not collect on it is, to us, a carnal sin.

Men have been having orgasms for as long as there have been men. Women on the other hand may or may not have had that luxury. Female orgasm is still a mystery to most of humankind. It does not have to be this furtive secret anymore and fortunately the cat is out of the bag now. With the global communication possibilities that now exist I boldly predict that it will become the norm rather than the unusual and iffy occurrence. We want to do our part to assist in the rapid spread of this information. A lot of the information that we will now describe can be useful in doing and seducing a man as well. So then why wouldn't every woman offered a do-date say "yes" to this proposal?

Explaining So You Can Be Doing

If necessary, explain what doing is and how you will put all of your attention on her while she will also put all of her attention on her pleasure and her orgasm—both of you at the same time focused on one orgasm. When people usually have sex or a sensual experience both people are trying to pleasure each other at the same time. This going back and forth between receiving and giving can be fun and is not something to give up for evermore. However, the divvying up of roles into giver and receiver or doer and doee can significantly increase the amount of pleasure that one potentially can feel. Doing is specifically utilized as a way to maximize the pleasure of each moment. It is an easier alternative for women to experience orgasm, as her clitoris will definitely be in play.

Basically, let her know that you will be using your hands to touch her. Your goal is to have her receive as much pleasure as she is able to. You want to relate this to her but not to create any pressure for her to have to perform or surpass any milestones. Let her (or him as this is true for either sex) know that she can take off as much of her clothes as she likes. At some point however to get the full effect she will have to take the risk and uncover her genitals to becoming exposed. You will keep your clothes on unless she prefers otherwise. All she has to do is lie there and feel. It would be great if she acknowledged moments that felt good to her but not to feel obligated to do so, especially in the beginning. Let her know in advance that you will make it as safe for her as possible by reporting what you will be doing before doing it and while doing it. You can also tell her in advance that you will be observing her body's responses and your own body's responses in relation to her and giving her feedback on what it is that you notice.

You are there to please her. In addition, you will take pleasure from giving her pleasure. She does not owe you anything in return for what you are giving her.

Another part of doing someone is to inform her that she can request whatever kind of stroke or pressure that she likes and if she does not know exactly to allow you to experiment with different strokes and pressures to determine what she does prefer.

Let her know that it is preferable to be as relaxed as possible while getting done and to refrain from helping by moving her hips or tensing up. It is possible to do somebody and allow them to be tensed up, but the relaxed way is preferable. We have found that the relaxed state is the one in which the body can experience extended orgasms naturally. Many people are used to tensing up while reaching for an orgasm and that is something that you can play with while you are doing them; for example, I will tell a woman to deliberately "tense up now" or to "relax now" so that they can feel their bodies more.

If she does not want any specific thing done or does not like something that you are doing; to let you know as soon as possible by please speaking up. In order to have it be as much fun as potentially conceivable for her she will benefit by getting her preferences met.

It is also a good idea to set up a time limit in the beginning. Fifteen minutes can be a good starting amount. If she and you want to continue longer than that then you both should agree to whatever extension you wish to add. She can always call it quits at any time she has had enough even if it is before the fifteen minutes are up.

Before beginning it is a good practice to ask her if she has any questions or would like any clarifications on any issues. You don't have to discuss all the matters that I have outlined as long as she understands what you are going to do and that she feel good about proceeding.

The Pussy as a Bargaining Chip

She believes if she has a sexual or sensual relationship with you that includes doing that you will not respect her or value her. This is some old puritanical thinking and she will hopefully have more than one viewpoint on this issue. Depending on how deep the roots of her negative prejudices are on the subject will determine if it is possible or how much work it will take to convince her otherwise.

Your intentions are not to cause her any harm but to have some fun. Doing will not give her any diseases or unwanted pregnancy. Will she be shamed in front of her family or friends for messing around with some man? Do they have to find out about it? What exactly is it that she is bargaining to get in exchange?

The fact is that people are viewpoint holders and are not their viewpoints and can have a number of viewpoints on many issues. She on the other hand may believe strongly that she is her viewpoint of religious indoctrination and think that having pleasure for pleasure sake is wrong. You will have to decide if it is worth it to pursue with your offer further.

This is where some of the seduction skills that we will talk about shortly can come in handy. Let her know that she does not have to do this now or ever for that matter. This is about pleasure for pleasure's sake and you can inform her that you understand that some people have a difficult time with that concept. By getting done it does not mean that you either must have an ongoing relationship or that it precludes having one. Because of her value system she may have to be in some kind of relationship with you already before any sensual pleasure is appropriate. Is that something that you are okay with?

She is thinking, "What Will I Owe for This?"

Tell her in advance that you get a lot of pleasure from doing this, that you have learned how to touch for your own pleasure and that she does not owe you anything in return. Giving a woman pleasure and gratifying her is one of the most fun activities that a person can do. If you are one of those guys who wants tit for tat and does not really enjoy pleasuring a woman then either learn how or pass on this whole subject. I know for myself that I do not require any reciprocation. If a woman has desire to pleasure you back it is not because she owes you anything but because she takes her own pleasure from doing so. It has to be real and don't allow her to do so if you think that she is doing it for any other reason. I don't want anybody touching me if she is not having a lot of fun when she does.

Sometimes one of the partners is always doing and the other one is always receiving. This is appropriate if everybody is on board with this, however, if it is too lopsided, it may become a problem. We have noticed that some women who have not had much in the way of orgasm in their lives when they finally learn how will want a strict diet of it until they have had their fill. You can feel fortunate that they have chosen you as the one who gives it to them. At some point they will feel filled up enough so that they can include more cock in their diet.

It is also good for them to know eventually that their orgasms and reception of pleasure will increase with their additional ability to offer this kind of pleasure. The better they progress in giving pleasure will allow them to receive that much more when they are getting done. It is helpful in becoming a better receptor of pleasure, as you get to see the experience from a different vantage point. We think that adding on different nuances when it comes to learning how to come better are all valuable. Talking with friends, watching others come or taking a class can all be beneficial.

To sum this section up, there are no sexual debts or obligations incurred if someone offers you pleasure.

They are Full (Sensually Speaking)

This is just another opportunity to play. Maybe she has been done so much that she is sore? This is probably not the case if she used lubricant and had a good partner. Sometimes a woman or a man who has had a lot of pleasure and has not acknowledged it can open himself or herself up for more fun by verbally appreciating the fun that they already had. By verbally acknowledging and writing or speaking your gratitude, a whole new vista of pleasure can become available.

Sometimes a person just has had enough; like too much of anything even fun and such delights as chocolate can become temporarily repellant. Hey, there is always tomorrow. The fact is that too much food or chocolate will make you feel sick a lot faster than sensuality via touching. Being sensually pleasured may have a limit but can also be returned to fairly quickly if you know what you're doing. This is another example why it is usually best to quit before someone is maxed out. If a person does not wish to be touched genitally there are countless other places and ways to give pleasure. Talking. Walking. Dessert.

Too Tired or a Headache?

These and similar responses are just resistances that men and women have and can potentially be removed if you are willing to put in the time and energy that it requires. They may or may not be true.

You know in your heart that it is possible to have pleasure, even a lot of pleasure, when you are tired or when you have some pain. Your resistant partner knows this too somewhere in the back of their mind. It's possible they want you to buy their excuses; they may want more caring, not less. Their resistance may even be a cry for help, figuring if you are not up to the challenge, it would be better for you to leave them alone.

We knew a couple in which the woman would resist pleasure by getting migraine headaches. We are not saying that the headaches were not real, but we learned she did use them to avoid intimacy with her partner. We suggested that he give her lots of loving attention, offer her a neck massage or a foot massage and just listen to her without trying to fix anything. She really liked this new way of just being allowed to feel the way she did without his resisting and fighting it. She relaxed more and after a while her desire for further sexual intimacy increased. She still got headaches, but together they used them to become closer and have some joy instead of fearing them as a deterrent.

By putting your attention on your distressed partner and not responding in kind to their negative demeanor you will have begun to melt the ice of resistance. They are not being in present time. They are losing about the past or the future either physically, emotionally, or both. They are in a state of victimization and pain, which is what spiritual teacher and author Eckhart Tolle would call their egoic mind and the pain-body. By you staying present and being as playful as the situation allows, you will offer them a better way to be. Just holding their hand and listening to them without arguing back will bring them closer to feeling better. As I said it may take some energy and lots of love to get them to agree to pleasure.

Sometimes it might be too much work and if they insist on leaving them alone, it might be a good idea to do so. Most importantly, you don't have to lose just because they are. Stay present and joyful and you will find that your presence will have a positive effect on your partner.

Nice Girls Don't

"Nice" girls do it, but they don't want to be too obvious or apparent at all in seeming to want to do it. So what is this it that they seem to recoil from? Here we are writing about getting done but it could be any form of sensual pleasure and it depends on the woman so it could be anything from first base to a home run, to revisit a metaphor popular in the mid-twentieth century. I googled this baseball reference and there was a wide discrepancy about what each base stood for. For example, some even had a fifth base for anal sex and others included that in third base or home base.

In any case they want you to take the seducer's role and then succumb and be the victim to your overwhelming desire. This way they can have their cake and eat it too. We are calling them nice girls, but how nice is it really to hold out pleasure from the universe? It is just their conditioning and society's pressures that have people act the way they do. We all want pleasure but imagine a universe where everyone was gung-ho about spreading the fun. Then again, all this fun we can have with seduction would no longer be necessary . . . so, it's a pretty good universe after all.

Resists Pleasure Chronically

Some religions and cultures consider female sexual pleasure sinful, something that corrupts the moral fiber of person who is supposed to be an honorable wife and mother. Growing up with that believe can taint a woman's perspective on pleasure forever.

Another scenario is that she may have had some bad experiences in the past and rather than chance a repeat of those has given up on having sensual pleasure.

By putting your attention on her and by asking pertinent questions you can find out specific resistances. Just the act of your interest in her will create an environment of increased trust and openness. Remember to keep your attention on her as you do not want to probe too deeply if she shows signs of resistance to that. Be playful and curious not like you are interviewing someone for a job. You can always come back to the sore spots later on after you have made some progress in other areas.

No to Naked; Bad Body Image

You obviously have not concluded your partner is unattractive or you would not desire her in the first place. Here you have to uncover the specific negative thoughts she is carrying around. Does she think that she is too fat? Too hairy? Is there only a specific part of her that she feels is unattractive? If you have enough attention on her you should be able to figure it out without having to inquire too intensely. It is time to flatter her. Tell her how beautiful she is, how you love her body and the way she smells. You can touch her through her clothes to get her aroused and desirous. You can perhaps have her expose small areas of her body at first. You can make it into a game that she actually has to leave some clothes on at first before you will allow her to do the full Monty.

A great exercise that works to help men and women learn to love their body is to spend some time in front of a mirror and look at themselves with loving eyes. Recommend this exercise to do alone and/ or together where you each take turns in front of the mirror. Usually when we look in a mirror, we look for things that are wrong with our body. In this exercise the goal is to find what we like and to approve of that.

Start with the easy parts that you can really approve of. You can even say out loud what it is that you like for example; "I love my eyes."

"I love my fingers." "I love my neck" Look at and comment on whatever it is that you like including your genitals. You will find more and more areas that you approve of. If you keep doing this, you will eventually fall in love with your whole body including the scars and the warts. The more you really like and start approving of your body the more it will actually change to be more beautiful. The more you like yourself the more sex appeal you will develop. You will feel more radiant and other people will notice that and respond to you differently.

The Non-existent or Rare Orgasm

This is a great opportunity, a chance to be a hero. Everyone wants to have pleasure, even though it is defined and described in different ways. If something is fun and safe, then almost everyone would say "yes" to it. Let her know that your viewpoint is that sensuality is about feeling whatever sensation is present. It is not about getting to any place but being there already at each moment. I have encountered many women who thought they were unable to have an orgasm. They would admit to feeling some pleasure in their past sexual lives but felt that they were inadequate and did not match up favorably to their sisters.

A big difference between you and me is that they came to us in order to find their sensual beingness and in your case they are still being reluctant about this desire. The probability though is that they would love it if someone were to deliver on this deficiency, though it is really a misconception. So, by explaining that whatever they are feeling is perfect and the way to expand this sensation is to approve of it just the way it is. All they have to do is put all of their attention or as much of it that they can on wherever you are touching them and approve of any good feelings that are occurring. It is likely that their focus will vacillate between feeling and thinking. As soon as they realize that they are thinking to put their attention back on their feeling just like in a meditation.

When you get good at doing you will be able to notice when your partner is feeling and when they are in their mind and have stopped feeling. If you can stop stroking her (or him) before she realizes she has lost focus, you will be in a great position to manage her orgasm. If you can stay one step ahead of her, then you will know exactly when to peak her. Trust your intuition. If you have the thought, "Maybe I should take a break," you definitely should take a break or relate something because you already are into thinking and have stopped feeling. Either take that break or communicate what you are noticing. This is an indication that she probably has gone into a similar mode. If you can notice that before she does you are getting closer to leading her into that dance of pleasure.

By being very approving and complimentary you will allow your partner to open up and be more present with their pleasure and their orgasm.

Measuring Up

This is similar to the last resistance covered. She is afraid that you won't enjoy her because she knows that you have done other more experienced and sensually trained women. To you it is an opportunity to have fun and that is the best approach to take with her too. You can start by talking to her. She is already into her head and her fear is proof that she is thinking and not feeling. Let her know how much you really desire her. Describe how sensuality is about feeling the pleasure now and not comparing yourself to anyone else. Tell her that you want her to feel her genitals. When you make this suggestion do so with your full intention. Help her get out of her head and focus on the pleasure that is already there. Get her into present time. Whenever she finds herself thinking or worrying to focus back on her pussy because that is what you will be doing also. You will be her co-conspirator for fun, and this is exactly where you want to be and what you want to do.

You can tease her. You can inform her that you will only touch her as long as it is fun to do so. Tell her to enjoy the breaks between the peaks and between the strokes. Again, let her know that all she has to do is appreciate whatever is happening at any one moment. She does not have to get to any place to be with pleasure. You can convey to her that you are not here to judge her but only to enjoy her.

The Lure of Seduction

This is really the prime resistance. All the other ones fall somewhere in here. Seduction is alluring for just about everyone. Men are usually less resistant and obviously have less at stake when saying yes, although that is mostly due to the possibility of coitus. They still enjoy being seduced. It is also the case that a female human can turn up her heat at will and many heterosexual males will capitulate easily to her will in this regard. I guess one could say that turn-on is a direct form of seduction. Some guys are more resistant and if a woman is not ready to use her trump card of turn-on she can still have fun seducing her partner by using her attention and wiles.

The most significant aspect to seduction by a male or a female is to enjoy the resistances that are presented. Understand that seduction is a game and have fun playing with the situations. I think that we can safely say people really want pleasure if they think they could have it safely and without any side effects.

Notice your partner when you make the offer of what you would love to do them. You can see by looking at them what their response is and be ready to shift directions quickly. By directions, I mean that if their answer is "no," then see it and raise them a bigger "no." We call this push/pull, so pulling is the offer and pushing is giving them a reason why they should not take your offer. Then when they come back towards you, you can counter your opposition with a counter reason why your objection is not really valid and that the opposite is the case. You are back to the pull.

For example:

Push: "I guess you are right. Doing can be very dangerous and harmful. Since I would be rubbing on you for an extended time it could hurt and cause abrasion."
Pull: "I will be very gentle and use lubricant when I touch your erogenous areas. It is very safe and you will feel only pleasure and wellbeing."
Push: "You probably are right you should not get done because you could become addicted to pleasure and you then

won't want to do anything else and you will become lethargic, lose your job and become homeless."

Pull: "In actuality, the people who I know that have more sensual pleasure in their lives are more creative and successful than the rest of the population."

These are obviously some general ideas. When it is your turn to create a push/pull procedure you can get more specific, basing them according to your partner's resistances and values.

At some point of your relentless attention you will feel your target's opposition wavering and their resistance weakened enough for you to start telling them what you want them to do and how to respond to you properly. This is when you can tell them to take their clothes off and to lie down naked.

Seducing Your Spouse or Regular Partner

Seducing your regular partner can be a challenge and again the first priority is to have fun with resistance. The added challenge is that she or he knows what you are up to and knows your lines. This is not a reason to give up because she really wants pleasure just as much as anyone else. So it is a reason to be more creative, more playful. Sometimes with Vera I will just set up the space with the towels and pillows on the bed. I put on some of her favorite music and I may then take her hand and lead her to the bedroom. I then hold her close to me in a sensual embrace and slowly kiss her on her neck and gradually make it to her lips. I can often feel her getting turned on by my antics: that is there is a stirring in my loins. Then I might say "Okay. You are really turning me on. You feel so good to hold. You have the best lips for kissing in the world. They are like a soft fluffy pillow with delicious overtones. Now I desire you to take off your pants." Amazingly this play works most of the time. Don't do the exact same trick every time. Be creative with a little variety so maybe kiss her in a different room first before you bring her to the bedroom. Tell her how sexy and beautiful she is. Maybe tell her that you are not going to do her. Have fun and let each moment of the seduction be the one that counts because that is a fact. If you don't make it to the doing part, you will have enjoyed whatever part you did do. More than likely, you will get her on the bed and she will let you play with her glorious glories.

I have often asked Vera over our many years together, simple questions such as: "Do you want to get done?" Would you like to be done?" or even "Can I do you?" or "Would you like me to do you?" The answer surprisingly to me for many years was usually no or not now or later dear. The question is kind of a set up to lose. Instead, I have found out the simple instructions: such as "Take off your pants" or "You are so beautiful and sexy, I want to have my way with you now" are more productive than the "friendly" questions.

The real answer to those questions is; "Of course I want to get done, dummy, but you are going to have to show me a little more desire and thoughtfulness before I surrender and say 'yes'."

It is similar when a woman asks a man, "Do you want to get done?" Of course, is the natural answer but it really does not matter what the words are but how she makes you feel when she claims that she wants to pleasure you. The most effective tactic is to turn up the intensity—to feel the intention behind the words. Instead of asking a question, start by having me feel her. Tell me to take my pants off or do it for me. Tell me to get undressed and lie on the bed. These words together with the even more important turn-on are what are going to make a fun seduction. I'm not saying that you should never use a polite question, but just that it is more effective to be playful.

Both men and women want pleasure, but we want to be overwhelmed and to be pleasure victims, to be the effect of someone else's desires. "It was not my fault he/she made me do it." There is a time and a place perhaps for the polite question but more often than not taking action with intention is far more effective. There is also a fine line between being pleasurably aggressive and raping someone and you have to respect each person's boundaries. A no means no. You can play with resistances if it is being fun for them too. If you notice that they are not enjoying your attentions, then back off whether with an old buddy or someone new.

You do have to be aware of your partner's tells, listen to them but, more importantly, watch their physical responses. You do that by keeping your attention on your partner and by reading their face and their body language, which is essentially more significant than what they are saying. I mentioned it earlier and repeat it now because it is vitally noteworthy. You have to enjoy the resistances and obstacles that are going to be there and if you are unable to have fun with them then it would be best to skip the whole process.

Undeserving of Pleasure

Here is where you can use some of your seduction skills. A lot of us grew up with the screwed notion of having to "pay" for pleasure. What exactly is the currency people who are not in the sex trade use to pay for pleasure? Unfortunately, it's with some form of pain or labor. How much pain is appropriate to allow you to feel that you finally deserve some fun? Who determines that someone is not deserving of pleasure?

Much of the world holds the viewpoint that sexual pleasure is somehow sinful. It inundates most of our lives to some extent. We called this underlying belief the *Pain Oriented Society* in our first book. We live in a world of mixed messages. It is agreed upon that sex sells. It just is not condoned to be the purchaser or the consumer of pleasure without having to have paid with some form of pain first. The example we used before which is still true today perhaps more so than ever in the United States is how much one has to work to feel entitled or even be allowed to take some time off for fun. How many hours a day does one have to work? How many days a week? How many weeks in a year? How many years before one can retire and do what one wants? All of these seem to be getting longer and not shorter. How many retired people are really enjoying themselves?

I am not complaining, which does not help anyway. I was just noticing and reporting the way things appear. Anyhow back to the seduction. This is an opportunity to tease them into saying, "Yes!" You can push them by making some kind of a remark about how they don't deserve having pleasure now and maybe not for a long time coming. They will buy that at first but then immediately reverse that logic.

You can also articulate how her having fun and a good time will make the universe a better place—at least your universe. The best person she can be is a joyous and happy one not someone who is losing and miserable. Bring her into present time where the focus will be on the moment at hand and not on what did or did not happen previously. If that first gambit does not work right away keep playing the game until resistance weakens and then just start with some form of sensual pleasure.

The Prerequisite of Love

Some people do feel that love must be present to have sexual relations. It is their conditioning and if it is so ingrained it will be difficult to sway them to another viewpoint. It also could be they are trying to avoid intimacy with you in particular.

Don't force yourself on anyone. It has to be fun for you and for them. You can be so much fun that they do fall in love with you or you can always move on.

Find out how far they will go. Will they accept a back massage? A foot rub? How intimate a kiss? Where do they draw the line? What is too intimate? For some people it will be intercourse while for some others it may be any genital exposure and stimulation. How about through the clothes? Once you know what their limits are you can play with those. Get close to the limit and back away. Show them that you can be trusted not to pass over their limitations. You can play push/pull by perhaps showing greater restraint than they are prepared to put up so that they will want to come towards you more. At some point they will learn to trust your integrity and allow you further intimacy.

Time Victims

I knew a woman who was very busy and would never make a date for pleasure. She did however like it on occasion to go for it on the spot, right then and there. That worked for me. You have to know whom you are dealing with. Some people, often couples, are so involved with their children that they believe they have no time for sensual pleasure with each other. If they want a more pleasurable life, they will have to be more deliberate about their schedule and priorities. Simple solutions like getting a sitter or going to a hotel room for one evening can be planned. Do what it takes.

If finances are a problem, which is another resistance, then create a special place like your own bedroom that does not have to cost anything where you won't be disturbed. It may just be a few minutes in the morning before the kids awaken if you are too tired at night. It could be getting grandma or grandpa to take the kids to the park for an hour on a weekend. With a little deliberate planning you can make pleasure happen. As we fully explained in our *Instant Orgasm* book, pleasure can be something done for a few seconds at a time whenever you please. It is available whenever you put your attention on it.

Perceived Incompetence

This time it is not the recipient, but rather the provider of pleasure who is thought not to measure up. Here is where it would be nice to have confidence and be ever the playful seducer. It is true that it would help if you were truly confident and if you were more knowledgeable about the female body and how to pleasure her. Perhaps it would be a good idea if you studied the subject. Meanwhile, you obviously are studying this matter if you are reading this; act like you do know something and let your playful side take over and enjoy the challenge.

It Wasn't Fun in the Past

This is similar to our last topic except the resistance is based on previous poor performances. Many married couples fall into this category as they once may have had a fun and a loving relationship but have acquired negative feelings and baggage with their partners over the years. There can be anger toward one another and the reality of not having developed any sensual skills. They may lack in knowledge of the different and varied activities that are available. There may have been sexual chemistry in the beginning that they did not require any additional skills to have a good time but with the loss of this chemistry things have just gone downhill. Instead of trying to enrich their sensual lives they have given up and either seek intimacy elsewhere or not at all.

The first part of the remedy is to admit that you have gotten to this stage. Then forgive yourself and each other. The second part is to realize that the past has no power over the present, as Eckhart Tolle likes to say and that you can start with a fresh attitude, like this being the first day of the rest of your life. If you have never done each other before in the manner that we describe or taken a class from the many coaches that are now out there, then there is a whole new vista of opportunity that awaits you. You can also do virtual classes by joining or buying videos from us or from the Welcomed Consensus or from Morehouse. Whichever path you take, they can all help you and your partner end in a good place if you both decide to make pleasure a priority. Learn how to give and how to receive great orgasmic pleasures. By staying in present time and enjoying this journey you will be creating a marvelous future for yourselves. You don't have to do this all at once. Take your time and enjoy this journey, as that is the only real way to take it.

Both members of a couple have to be on board for this renewal to work. Otherwise, it would be best to get a new partner unless you can really develop your seduction skills. It is easy to say drop the anger and the old withholds but it can be difficult for some people to actually accomplish. We have dealt with the topic of anger before but basically anger is something you choose whether consciously or not. If you do decide to take the healthy route you will be well rewarded.

The Physical Turn-Off

Some people have developed some repulsive habits over their years. Some people are just repulsive to a specific group of people. Sometimes it is best to walk away from someone who finds you revolting. Other times it may be a good idea to find out what it is that they find revolting about you and do something about it. I would guess that often a person's repulsiveness would have more to do about how they feel about themselves than actually about their beingness. So if this is happening every time out with different potential partners maybe it is time to start loving yourself more. In order to ask someone to do them, they are obviously already in your association. They must like you enough to be around you.

Take your yucky attention off of yourself and start noticing who it is that you would like to become more intimate with. Use the seduction skills covered above. Enjoy their resistances. A lot of not so attractive men are with beautiful women and vice versa. Don't take yourself or the situation too seriously. All you want to do is to give them some pleasure by doing them. You can tease them about how you just might just turn into a handsome prince if they let you put your froggy hands upon their garden.

Is Doing Considered Sex?

A friend asked me that question recently. I said yes and no. According to the dictionary, doing is not considered sex. For something to be considered sex there has to be the possibility of procreation with a male gamete and a female gamete. But that would make anything other than penis into vagina including oral, anal or hand or any kind of things not sex. That would make playing with inanimate objects in a pleasurable way not sex.

Orgasm is about pleasure and one can have it with a partner or on one's own with or without touching. This depends on one's ability to feel and the extenuating circumstances. We have met some people who are able to just feel their bodies expansively and have their energy flow so that they can have an extensive orgasm without touching. They usually have trained to do this, and it appears to be challenging to control.

In my view orgasm including self-pleasuring, doing, any kind of sensual touching are all sexual activities and therefore I consider them to be sex. So here I have answered the question: yes, doing is sex. The home run to me is any activity that produces great pleasure and intense orgasm. In baseball there is a saying especially in the late innings that a walk or a small hit is just as good as a home run. The analogy here is that you don't have to go for the big orgasm or big home run; just feel as much as you can at this moment, which is really the only thing that you can do.

Then again if the person that you are seducing resists the idea of having sex with you because they are waiting till being married or until they know you better, you can tell her that you are not going to have sex with her; that you just want to do her and doing is not sex.

We have given you a number of possible resistances and how to handle them. The next chapter will delve into creating more intimacy with better communicating when giving and receiving pleasure. Some of these skills that you will be learning will also make you a more confident and better seducer.

5

Sexual Communications

In this chapter we will present you with some ideas on how to up your communication skills in bed and elsewhere. We will describe the importance of using words to acknowledge your pleasure and the benefits of connecting your throat to your orgasm. We will explain how to take control of your partner's nervous system by using your attention to your partner, fantasy, and expression.

Verbalizing in Bed

"Ooh ahh" is a start but it is not enough if you are serious about upping your quality of lovemaking. You will have to learn to speak while either giving or receiving an orgasm.

The most important aspect of orgasm is to feel. If you are engaging your mind instead of your tactile sensations, you will be missing part of the experience depending on how much clutter is going on in your mind. Therefore, it would seem that not thinking and not speaking might be your answer. This would be too simplistic and remove some of the possible fun and pleasure from your experience. Not speaking is what a lot of people have been doing anyhow because of our conditioning not to speak while having sex. I recently saw a comedian on television and he was making fun of people who wanted to talk when having sex. Paraphrasing here, he said the only time he will say anything while having sex is if a big rig was about to crash into them.

There is a line and I don't think it is too fine between not talking enough and talking too much. Most people fall into the not talking enough category hence learning how to talk while sexing will be our emphasis. You also want to keep the conversation on what you are doing. To talk about other things such as gossiping about folks or about business issues when doing or getting done is counter-productive. This does not mean that you can't have some fun dialogue about unrelated issues if it brings the two of you joy. It is fine to talk a little about other things once in a while just not to do that very frequently and probably best to take a break from the touching when doing so.

The trick or answer that we have found that works best in learning how to communicate while sexing is to hook up your sensations to your verbal output. Because of our conditioning not to speak, this ideal model will not be so easy for some folks. It will probably take practice and training. Since practicing and training are what we expect you will be doing anyhow, adding better communication skills to your sensual life will only help.

Mind Wandering

The goal is to communicate verbally and at the same time not to think too much or delve into your mind while you are receiving or for that matter producing pleasure in your partner's body. You do not want to be thinking too hard about what to say but you do want to be saying something to your partner about the pleasure that you are receiving. This gets easier and easier the more you practice it; if at first you get distracted by your mind interfering with your pleasure chalk it up to a necessary exercise to gain strength of your pleasure facilities. It is kind of like in meditation when you are focusing on your breathing or attempting to stop the chatter of your mind.

The wandering and continual thoughts of our minds has generally become the normal state for most people, as John Kabat Zinn explains in his *Mindfulness* approach. All one has to do is to notice that you started your compulsive thinking again and then go back to putting your attention back on your breathing, for example.

So having a great sexual experience or a "power of now" (to use Eckhart Tolle's words) sensual experience is to be there fully for the pleasure. As soon as you notice that you have started mind wandering and doing mental masturbation, just focus attention back to the pleasure that is right there in front of you. Again, don't beat yourself up for something that everyone does and that you have been conditioned to do. In all likelihood, your partner will duplicate your mind wandering and you both will disappear from the experience together. The trick is to come back to the pleasure as soon as you notice that you have left. You can even communicate to your partner how you are back now. This may be a good time for a break from the physical experience, especially if the wandering was prolonged. This way you can communicate what just happened and how you both feel. You can then start up again with the physical pleasuring. A person receiving pleasure will be thankful that you noticed the mind taking a break away from the present moment. They can relax and surrender more effortlessly knowing that you have your attention on them.

A lot of this chapter deals with the abilities and communication skills necessary to manage your partner's orgasm. The better you are at communicating, the easier it will be for your partner to give up the controls to you, or what we call surrendering their nervous system. Control in the sense that we use it here is a positive attribute. It has no relationship to acting like a control freak.

Communication Lags

If you do not communicate well, you will make a lousy lover. If you communicate too slowly in response to someone else's communication, it will be indicative of what kind of lover you are. It is also indicative of what kind of person you can be. Not responding to someone's communication or inquiry in or out of bed in an appropriate time can be irritating and annoying. It is of course up to the person being annoyed or irritated what kind of response they will feel and their choice in the end; but also know that most people are not that conscious all the time and there will be some needless negativity created.

Looking at the out of bed scenario, this interaction can be in the form of an email, phone message, physical mail, text message or even a direct conversation or whatever kind of communication you are involved with. The better you are able to listen and respond to another person the less of a communication lag will be created. This will create good will and peaceful thoughts. On the other extreme the longer the lag the more negativity has a chance to build. Many people are so absorbed in themselves that they make poor listeners. When someone mentions something, the usual response is something like, "Me too," and then they go on to talk about themselves. Everyone wants to talk, and few people really want to listen to someone else. Heed the famous saying, "There is a reason that we have two ears and only one mouth." I have taken up the habit recently of using licorice lozenges sweetened with xylitol. There is a quotation on every box. One of them stated a quote by musician Jimi Hendrix, surprisingly to me of all people. "Knowledge speaks but wisdom listens." That sums it up nicely.

Sometimes a person receiving the message, whether verbal or otherwise, may not actually absorb the message for some reason. They are too busy talking or they are lost in their own mind clutter or an email was mistakenly sent to a spam folder or to a wrong address, and so on. This is why it also is important to check whether your communication got through if you are not getting an appropriate timed response. With today's electronic communication, that is simple to do. Imagine living just a couple of centuries ago and sending a letter and not hearing back. There was little you could do to ensure that your message was received.

Knowing the person who you are sending or trying to communicate with can help the communicator understand how much a communication lag one can expect. If the person is really busy juggling kids, work and life they may not get back to you as soon as you would like. However, I know many busy people who make it a point to answer their outstanding communications swiftly. I have had a number of doctors who either got to the phone right away or made sure to call back or have their nurse call back in a timely fashion. I have also had doctors who took a few days or even not call back at all to get back to me where I had to make several phone calls to get their attention. I did not keep those doctors who treated me like that. A good communicator will do better in any business as well as being a better lover.

Out of the bedroom or in it, it will benefit you to learn to communicate and acknowledge better. We have a number of grandchildren that we give small but not insignificant gifts to for Christmas and Birthdays. Some of them enthusiastically and quickly respond with thank you and appreciation. Some of them take a long time and others don't respond at all. It makes it a lot more fun to give to someone whether it is anonymously or even with strings attached to have it be appreciated. I know for myself that next Christmas or next birthday I will be inclined to gift those that were more appreciative with better gifts than the ones who were unappreciative. It is just human nature.

Getting back to the bedroom, almost. The better you become at communicating outside the bedroom, the more you will enhance your abilities inside the bedroom. It is vitally important to acknowledge your partner for any pleasure that you are experiencing that they are cause for or that is happening between the two of you. This can be pleasure received from your partner or pleasure you feel when you are the giver. The faster and more happily you can verbally appreciate any positive attention or sensations, the more you will elevate the pleasure significantly. As soon as you feel any bit of pleasure with your partner, acknowledge it right away before it slips away. Once you become comfortable with talking during sex, then speaking up will also keep you in the present moment instead of thinking about if or what you should be saying. We have noticed when people are pleasuring their partners that he or she may be rubbing them for minutes at a time without either one of them saying anything.

When the person doing receives positive appreciation from their partner, their attention will increase notably as they will feel good about what they are doing and will have the reinforcement to continue. It is so much fun to do someone who is appreciating your actions. A lack of verbal appreciation is a communication lag and can often turn a fun experience into a buzz kill. You can know for certain that almost everyone under-acknowledges the good or positive sensations as compared to complaining about the bad (again inside the bedroom and without). The more appreciative you are in bed and in any other circumstance will add more pleasure to your life and those around you.

Who's Talking?

This verbal acknowledgment can emanate from either the person receiving the pleasure or the person who is giving it. This verbal appreciation that I am describing is important for the divided roles of sexing or even if you are both giving and receiving at the same time. It is also usually contagious to express value for someone. The more and the better that you demonstrate how much fun you are having, the more you will instill in your partner a desire to behave similarly. Acknowledging them more and you will likely have that reciprocated.

As part of our training, we want our students to continually to be practicing approval. If it is difficult for them to verbally acknowledge their pleasure in bed we will sometimes assign them homework of expressing appreciation for a less-charged subject. This can be practiced while enjoying a tasty meal or just looking at themselves in front of a mirror. They can do it with their friends or even by themselves.

Connecting Sound to Orgasm

There is a way to connect your throat and the sounds that come from it to your orgasm. It just takes practice and noticing how your own voice can enhance the feelings in your body. Moaning and deep guttural sounds are probably easier to connect at first than regular words but with practice any sound that you make can deliver more pleasure.

Speaking of moaning, some people over-moan and some people don't moan at all. By over-moaning, I mean the little pleasure being produced does not match the big sounds and this can be a distraction. If the orgasm is a big one, then even loud moaning will feel right, and it won't be a distraction. We believe that moaning is a powerful tool that can help connect your orgasm with your throat and creating a full-body orgasm not isolated to your crotch.

It also can be a way some people avoid using words as they think that moaning is enough. It could be enough if you want to put a top limit on your pleasure but if you want to soar even higher, then the addition of words that are fully expressive of how you feel can help take you there. On the other hand, moaning and guttural sounds can be a fun addition to your pleasure if you are the quiet type who does not make a sound when having an orgasm. I have learned to make guttural or deep throat sounds to increase my sensation and even extend my peaks. It sounds like a deep "chaa" resonance coming out of my throat. It is similar to the sound you make when gargling only you don't have the water or mouthwash. Again, it is a good idea to experiment with different sounds to find one that resonates with your own body. I have seen many women increase their orgasmic pleasure with sounds from deep in their throat. One woman made sounds that sounded like a "whoa whoa whoa" repetitive moan from deep in her throat. Another woman used a sound like "ahh ahh ahh" to connect to her pussy. I have witnessed other women getting off well who are gasping as they have an orgasm. There are all kinds of vocal sounds that you can experiment with to see what fits best for you.

Sometimes under some circumstances such as trying to be surreptitious, perhaps in your parent's home, doing it quietly might be a good idea. Otherwise open your lungs, take some deep breaths and let the sound release. When you are in a deep state of orgasm, the sounds will extend the peak and can even take you to a higher precipice. I think it is a good idea to be behind closed doors but to be noisy enough so that your kids know that their folks are having a fun time. If while you were raising them you were quietly doing it for their entire lives and suddenly changed to becoming loudly vocal you probably should talk to them first about that so they will understand; otherwise, they will probably think it is weird, which they might think anyhow.

Overprotecting one's children seems to be common these days. Protecting them from dangerous things is fine to an extent. Protecting them from finding out that their parents are healthy sexual beings is senseless. I am of the opinion that young people would have a better adolescence if they knew about orgasm and how to self-pleasure. Orgasm is natural and fun. Having intercourse when too young is dangerous, however; if we were to have sex education classes in schools where masturbation and doing were taught competently, I believe we would have a more informed and healthier society.

Speaking Words

What words should you be saying while being pleasured? This is something that you will have to develop and create for yourself and your partner. Every one of us is unique and how we speak and what we say has to be real and genuine. You are not memorizing a script as in a play but letting authentic feelings express themselves. The more you practice the easier it will be for the words to just come out of you naturally. You do not want to be lying there and thinking of what to say. That will take you away from the orgasmic pleasure you were feeling. A sound suggestion is to keep it simple at first. There's no need to be grammatically correct. Short sentences with a few words or a couple of syllables will work. So utterances like "Yes!" "Wow!" "Oh yeah!" "Right there! "You got me!" are some examples. Feel the words and sounds coming forth from your throat and out of your mouth. Feel your genitals at the same time and you can build a connection between your voice and your orgasm. The more specific your words are will also enhance your experience. So "That spot on my clitoris, yes!" "Right there." "You hit the spot!" is better than saying "it all feels so good."

By combining some vocal sounds with occasional words while you are in an orgasmic state will generate a connection if practiced deliberately. Practice when self-pleasuring or with your partner. The more that you practice this, the easier it will become and your voice will flourish. We had an opera singer as a student a number of years ago and she learned to get off with her voice. It also made her singing besides being more fun for her to sing become stronger and more polished.

Snappy Patter

We have trained many people in the art of pleasuring women via hands on techniques. The ability to communicate while pleasuring your partner goes hand in hand with your hands. It is extremely beneficial to talk to your partner while you are doing them whether they are a man or a woman. One of the ways to come better is to acknowledge the pleasure that one is feeling. By acknowledging the pleasure that you are feeling in pleasuring your partner will enable your partner who is being pleasured to speak more freely and easily. Because of our conditioning to not speak while having sex it may feel a bit awkward to talk from either receiving or giving pleasure. The easier you make it for your partner to speak and acknowledge their pleasure the better lover you will become.

We also have noticed some men who we are training to pleasure their partner, moan and groan while doing so. This is not a good idea. You always want to maintain at least an illusion of control when giving pleasure and by moaning you will be demonstrating the lack of it. To sum it up, it is good to moan when receiving pleasure, not so good when you are giving it. That being said, I think that it is different if a woman is doing a man, though it might be my own sexism. If a woman is having orgasmic feelings and not faking it while pleasuring someone it might be a turn-on to their partner if she is moaning. (Then again, I get turned on by Maria Sharapova screaming as she hits the tennis ball.) It still is probably better if a woman used words and verbalized what she was experiencing when pleasuring her partner.

Positive feedback while you are stroking your partner or doing them can be helpful to them and to you. It keeps you focused on what you are doing. Again, you don't want to have to think too hard about what to say. Just say what you are feeling as your attention is on your partner. You don't want to lie. To lie is using up too much of your limited attention on thinking besides misleading your partner on how you are actually feeling. Use words that you feel comfortable with and that feel natural coming out of your mouth. I will give you some suggestions, but it is best if you make the words your own. So, for men or women doing the pleasuring here are some examples.

"You have a beautiful body."
"You are so sexy."
"Your skin is so smooth."
"It feels great to touch you."
"Your pussy is luscious."
"Your cock is throbbing."
"You're getting wetter and wetter as I stroke."
"Your contractions are getting stronger."
"Your penis feels so good in my hand."
"You are coming easy."
"Your clitoris is getting redder and bulbous."
"Your penis is so hard. It feels amazing."
"I can feel you inside."
"The peaks are getting higher."
"This is the best one yet."
"Your penis is so hot."
"Your pussy is so sexy."
"My pussy is throbbing from my touching your penis."
"Your pussy is really turning me on."
"I am hard as a rock."
"I love your thighs."

So, while you are focused on your partner's genitals, it really is their whole body that you can be pleasuring. It is a good idea to look at their face once in a while not always looking at their crotch. Sometimes people tense up their faces and that can be a giveaway to have them relax more. You can also look into their eyes and connect with them on a more personal level. It is a lot easier to tell what a person is really felling when you look at their eyes and face and not only at their crotch. A person receiving pleasure also feels that you are really noticing them if you look at them face to face. It is important to look at their genitals and notice what is happening down there but not to the detriment of ignoring the rest of the person. So some other things you can say as you gaze at their face are; "You look so beautiful." Your cheeks are really red and engorged just like your genitals." "Your face is glowing with ecstasy." "You look like the poster face for joy." "I love your deep delight." "You are radiating pure bliss." Some women may feel shy at first and close their eyes and not want you to look them directly in their eyes. Depending on how you feel you can accept this behavior, or you can use your seduction skills to get them to open up more. In any case this is an opportunity to communicate.

Connecting the Pussy to the Brain

In addition, some women who are new to getting done and being totally at effect will not have connected their pussy to their brains to the extent that will happen if they continue to practice. By look-ing at their face you will notice that even though their pussy is being orgasmic they are not feeling as much as they can or will. This is an opportunity to talk more, take a break and to communicate what is happening in their genitals. If you tell someone that her pussy is working beautifully but that you can tell that she is not feeling it all, she can surrender some more to you, realizing that you are right. By noticing your partner and communicating what is going on, you will be able to have them focus their attention on their pleasure. More breaks and shorter peaks with steady communication will be helpful to them to connect their genitals to their brains. It can help to go slowly and pointing out the individual contractions to strengthen the neural pathways. Recognizing your own orgasm can help you catch up to the orgasm you are already having.

You may not feel that the power button to your pussy is turned on when you first begin touching yourself. Keep at it. Be playful with yourself, take lots of breaks and just feel as much as you can at each individual moment. Your orgasms will seem to get better and better and more intense as you practice. You will no longer have doubts that your pussy is plugged in and that the energy is circulating.

Extending Orgasm with Words

One of our orgasmic techniques is to teach our students how to extend the orgasm. Noticing your partner's level or direction that the orgasm is being felt is important to succeeding at this endeavor. In order to extend the orgasm, you have to be able to predict whether the next stroke will be beneficial to increasing the pleasure or will it have your partner feel less pleasure. The more you pleasure someone the better you will become in being able to predict how to proceed. Trust your instincts. It is also better to peak them too soon than too late. If you were wondering whether the next stroke would take them higher or lower you are already in your head and have stopped feeling so, yes, it would be a good idea to take a break. The usual way to peak someone is to take a break or change the stroke. Another perhaps more unconventional way to peak them is to peak their interest by using your verbal abilities.

Instead of taking a break from stroking, sometimes you can coax them to go up by suggesting just that. You can say something like: "Keep feeling." "Feel it more." "Feel this stroke now." "Stay focused." Stay with me now." Or simply, "Take it up a notch." Or the warning, "I'm going to stop." Or "I'm going to take a break if you don't take it higher." As soon as you feel that you got their attention and their orgasm is back on track, let them know by acknowledging their response. You can say again simple words like "Perfect!" "I feel you stronger than ever." "You're flying."

That is also why it is so important to frequently give your partner positive feedback along the way. Otherwise, it would appear you are bullying in a way. If you previously just told her how great it feels touching her clitoris or that the contractions are getting stronger, then when you ask her to feel more, she will be more inclined to listen to you. By again acknowledging her after she's responded so well you have completed a valuable communication cycle.

When the response to your suggestion is in the positive direction, keep on stroking and acknowledging. However sometimes your partner will resist your encouragement and not respond so well. If you don't get a quick response to your verbal boost, then you will have to take her down and peak her by the regular way of stopping the stroke or at least changing it. Communicate to your partner what you are doing and what just happened. Then you can also ask questions to find out how she is feeling. You can ask straight out, "Have you had enough?" or "Do you want some more strokes?" Listen to the answer and how it makes you feel. Look at her face to see better what is going on with her. A person can say one thing, but the face will tell you the truth.

Sometimes a little coercion will allow your partner to start going up again. Other times, that's not so, but you want to be sensitive to what your partner really wants so they can trust your feelings even more the next time. The person getting done always can go for more with real desire. Maybe they just required a longer break. Their desire is easily picked up and noticed and you can always start again if called upon with some real aspiration.

Also, if this is a new person that you are pleasuring remind them before you touch them that you may give them some suggestions while stroking them such as "Relax!" or "Feel more!" or "Push out." and that they do not have to judge these promptings or think about them at all. All they have to do is to have their bodies listen and without the mind filter, their bodies will respond accordingly.

A push out is where the person receiving the orgasm pushes out their sphincter muscles as if they are going to defecate and urinate at the same time. It is the opposite of tensing up or pulling in of these muscles and is a technique that helps them relax. Hopefully, they have peed before they started and there will not be any accidents. Also, the push out is only for a second or two so this should not cause any problems. After the quick push out, they continue to stay relaxed.

Sometimes we will even say things such as; "If you don't talk to me, I am going to stop stroking." "I know that you can feel more." "Fill up the room with your orgasm." "Take it up another level." These are said in a loving and friendly way and can produce the desired results, which you can then acknowledge with approval as soon as they respond accordingly. Different people respond to different types of words. Some people like it all sugar coated and others like it tough and direct. Most people fall somewhere in between. Know whom you are dealing with and choose your words accordingly.

More About Extending the O

To extend the orgasm in both men and women, you have to become familiar with the bodily responses that your partner is experiencing while you are pleasuring them. That means that your attention is focused on them while you are touching them. It also means that the more you practice with them the better you will be able to read their orgasm. It helps to train with the same partner so that their orgasmic cycles of up and down is recognizable to you. Everyone has a different yet similar pattern so practicing in general will afford you greater clarity on the direction of an orgasm. At some point in your training this ability to recognize where your partner's orgasm is headed will become like second nature to you and your own body will know exactly what to do and when; bypassing your thinking process almost entirely.

Basically, what you are basing their orgasm on and how your orgasmic prediction is made is by noticing how you are feeling in relation to the pleasure they are demonstrating. That is another reason why it is easier to control someone's pleasure levels with your hands than with your genitals or mouth. You are feeling the contractions and at the same time feeling the pleasure in each stroke that you are giving them. If you were to keep stroking someone no matter how well you are doing it, there will come a point where the pleasure will either plateau or decrease. The goal is to peak them deliberately before the sensation decreases or the plateau is no longer as much fun as it was. Also, at times, especially when you are new to this game, your awareness of the pleasure will tend to fluctuate and will even tune out altogether and you will be reflecting about something else that your mind just happened to think about. In any of these scenarios the best course of action is to take a break.

Taking Control

A lot of what I've been just writing about are ways that a pleasure producer or doer can implement taking control of their partner's orgasm. As we have repeatedly stated the goal of the pleasure receiver is to surrender their nervous system. Therefore, the person who is providing the pleasure has to do what it takes so their partner can surrender. One of the ways that this is accomplished is by what we call "safeporting." Safeporting is just a fancy term for creating a space that feels safe and puts the person who is being done in a position of less vulnerability. To be receiving the pleasure where the most fun is possible is also the most risky position. You want to lower this vulnerability as much as you can so that the receiver of your attentiveness can put all their attention on their pleasure and not have to worry or wonder about external interruptions or unexpected occurrences. Simply informing them of what you will be doing next and describing any unusual disturbances that can crop up can provide this safeporting.

So phrases such as "I am going to touch your clitoris now," "I am going to take a break now," o "I am going to put some lubricant on you," "That ringing is the phone and we are not going to answer it now," or "That's just the neighbor walking around upstairs," will help the recipient of your attentions to trust you to be in control of the situation and allow them to have another reason to surrender. You can also communicate how you are going to use more pressure or less pressure or a faster or slower stroke as well as any other changes you will be doing. Surprise is usually a cause for going down and a way to lose control. There may be times when you want to use surprise to get someone's attention but in general communicating what you are up to is the best way to stay in control. If you do space out and forget to use some safeporting like touching them without telling them first, then describe what you are doing as soon as you realize it. Don't dwell on any misses and put your attention on whatever you are doing or going to do next. As you probably realized by now, I like to use baseball analogies. If you are the batter and you just swung and missed a pitch, you have to focus on the next pitch coming up now, not on that last one or you will miss this one too.

Using Fantasy to Control

Some people enjoy fantasy when being stimulated sensually and other people could care less. If you know your partner well and know that they enjoy fantasy and what kind of fantasy they like you can use it to increase their pleasure. Some people enjoy fantasy so much that they are doing it secretively while you are pleasuring them. This is okay but it may be even more fun if you took control of their fantasy as well as their body.

Women usually have more of a story line to their fantasy and men tend to visualize sexy women or perhaps just a sexy body part. This is not always the case so again it is important to know your partner's likes and dislikes. They call it fantasy because it is of the imagination and not necessarily something that you actually want to happen though some fantasies you might not object to.

Some women may have a fantasy about being kidnapped by pirates and forced to have sex with more than one pirate at a time. She may just like to fantasize about the scenario and a description of the boat and what the pirates are wearing. Maybe she has them slowly take off her clothes and then they take off theirs. She might like to hear about how they fill all of her orifices at once with their engorged members or she may not even want to hear about any specifics. Find out what she likes best and use your imagination to take control of her fantasy thoughts while you are touching her.

Some women may prefer to have a fantasy in which they are in the dominant position and get to choose who gets to be with her like in a pornographic *Bachelorette*, or a fairy tale princess who has all kinds of suitors to choose from. A woman might fantasize about being on top while having intercourse or making a guy or guys sexually engorged from her beauty without having to touch them. We have known women who fantasized about other women or even about having sex with horses or other well-endowed animals. Fantasies are about adding more fun to your sensual life and we do not judge someone for wanting more fun no matter how unusual their imagination runs.

Men too can have fantasies about dominating or being dominated. It can be exciting to a guy for his partner to bring in an imaginary partner while getting done. Vera on a number of occasions would pick out a woman whom she knew I fantasized about and while stroking my penis would say things like, "Look here, Cindy from the gym just came into the room. She is wearing a real short skirt and is topless. She has amazing long legs. She has beautiful strong thighs, and she is putting your cock between them. She is squeezing your cock firmly with her strong thighs and then relaxing them and then squeezing them again over and over and over. You can't get away. Cindy's got you." While she is turning me on with the story, she is squeezing my cock in her hands to the same rhythm that "Cindy" is using and it feels so good.

A girlfriend of mine used her own imaginary body to stimulate my mind into erotic ecstasy. She said while doing me with her hands something like, "We are wrestling and I pin you down on the floor. I am having my way with you. My thigh is rubbing against your cock and you are my pussy prisoner. I am putting your cock between my strong calf muscles and dominating you. I am now getting on top of you and I'm fucking you really hard up and down and up and down. You are screaming for mercy and I don't stop. She is using her hands and controlling my penis as she is filling my head with erotic thoughts. She is doing me in synch with the story and it all feels so good.

Again, some guys like it when they are in charge in their fantasy and fantasize about being in the dominant position and making the woman squeal with delight from their thrusting while on top of them. If that is the case or any other kind of male dominant fantasy, then create a fantasy that will provide him with that kind of stimulation of his mind.

I have found that enjoyable sexual encounters with partners who used their imagination and that were extraordinarily fun are applicable to be re-fantasized when self-pleasuring. That is something that I have incorporated in my self-pleasuring and I presume probably works for a lot of other folks. A lot of people are ashamed of their fantasies as they feel that others will find them wrong for having "strange erotic ideas." They therefore do not tell anyone about them yet they continue to use them. They then often feel guilty for having such thoughts. It really helps to confide in your partner so you are not alone with these thoughts. If your partner finds you "wrong," perhaps they are the wrong partner for you. You don't have to write a book like I am doing and tell the whole world about your fantasy but at least your supposedly best friend can be included.

Attention Equals Control

To be in control is kind of a misnomer in that what you are actually doing is putting so much attention on your partner that they feel that you are more in touch with their body than they are themselves. So, to be in control does not have anything to do with bullying another person or making them do what you want. You are really serving them where they feel that they no longer have to spend energy to do any kind of work. They can lay back and just be. They can put all their attention on feeling the sensation that is occurring at that moment. They can surrender to the good feelings that you are producing. Their goal is to be total effect and by you taking the role of total cause they can realize their optimum orgasmic potential.

The specific attention that you are giving them is to notice exactly what would feel best at any given moment. It must feel good to you at the same time. The better you know your partner and more familiar with their desires the easier in some ways it becomes. You know what pressure they like, what kind of strokes feel best, and so on. You know if they like to have music, what kind of music. You know how high they like to have a pillow behind their head or a pillow under their legs. When you first start out with a new partner you have to learn all these things. The easiest way to find out is to ask them questions. Once you are familiar you can still ask questions from time to time but it won't be so frequently.

Each time you do the same person it will not be exactly the same as any other time. That is where your attention is vital so that you notice what is the appropriate act to do next. What will feel best? Sometimes you will avoid the genitals and clitoris for a long time and another time it may be fitting to go straight to the clitoris. Sometimes a woman may want some hand penetration from the start but usually she will prefer to be stimulated for a while before you do that. Sometimes a peak will last a long time and other times it will only be a few strokes. The same kind of attention will work when doing a man. Enjoy each stroke that you are giving with as much pleasure as you can feel. When you feel like taking a break, don't hesitate.

Taking a Break

Sensuality is about having the most fun and the most pleasure that you can have at any particular moment. It is a misnomer to call this sexuality but because of the common usage we will include that term too. To keep on stroking because of wanting to have a successful outcome is not about pleasure. Breaks are an equally important aspect of the pleasure cycle. Eckhart Tolle describes the importance of space in comparison to form in his books—and silence in contrast to sound. The break in the orgasmic form that is touch to include some space or not touching will intensify the orgasmic energy. It will inform your partner that your attention is on them and they will be more able to surrender their orgasm to you. It will allow them to feel more once you start touching them again. The break is the space that gives the touch its intensity.

There is no specific formula of when to take a break or when to start again. This will depend upon the orgasmic circumstances that are present. Sometimes when I am manually stimulating someone who is new to the experience, I may only stroke a couple of times before a short break and do this over and over until I feel that they will be able to keep feeling on the third stroke. Then I will feel what the length of the next peak will be and it may be only four strokes in a row with a break and do that a few times and so on until a steady dose of strokes will be appreciated and felt with rising intensity. I will communicate to them exactly what I am doing and letting them know when I will be starting up again, which could be almost immediately or not, depending on what I feel.

There are other scenarios where the woman has experience being done, or a newcomer is a natural and able to be present with every stroke that you are doing. Then just keep stroking her as long as the sensation is not fading. If your hand is tired take a break. If your mind starts to wander away from what you are doing, take a break. If you are thirsty take a break. If you have to go to the bathroom, take a break. All these are signs that your attention is no longer as potent as it was. It is not a sin to take a break when the orgasm is going well. It is a lot better than to keep stroking when it is not.

In the next chapters we will provide you with some specific touching techniques to provide you with a sturdy foundation that you can build on once you know what you are doing.

6

Giving Pleasure, Enjoying the Touch

This chapter and the next are about giving pleasure. Instead of separating doing women from doing men entirely I have blended the description together where it is possible. Then when it is necessary, I have divided and provided specific information on both the touching of female and male genitals. This first chapter is about teasing and arousing the focal points of the clitoris and the homologous area under the corona of the penis by touching elsewhere on their bodies. I then proceed with a thorough description on lubricating the genitals.

About to Touch

The first part of this chapter will be unisexual, that is, appropriate for touching a woman or a man. Then we will delve into the particulars and describe the way to touch a specific gender. If you have thoroughly read the previous chapter, we have presented to you quite a bit of communication skills. They will make the touching aspect of doing a lot easier if they are incorporated. We will continue to remind you about proper communications as we describe how to touch.

The first and perhaps most important aspect of touching someone else is that it has to feel good to you. The only real way of giving pleasure is by having pleasure. If the touch feels for any reason un-pleasant to you then you should not be touching that person at that moment.

This is true for all of your senses. If something is disagreeable either change it or get into agreement with it.

If the body odor of the person you are touching is displeasing to you then you should do something about that, too. Either have your partner wash, which would be my first choice, or spray something pleasant on them that overpowers the odor. (The latter would be a very Elizabethan way to go.) If it is your regular partner who usually smells fine, but this time does not, then it will be no problem to ask them to clean up. If it is someone you are having sex with for the first time, then you will have to handle it delicately with proper communications and support. You might suggest showering together as a start. If their genitals have too strong an odor for you, just ask if they could wash up down there before you begin. Some people prefer a strong odor and some prefer it squeaky clean. Also, we have noticed that some women who are fearful about having all the attention on them will give off a bit of an odor associated with this fear. Once you start stroking, it usu-ally goes away quite quickly or maybe one just does not notice it after a while. In any case if something bothers you, make sure that you take care of it in a nice way.

If your partner has some rash or herpes sores on their genitals, this too has to be handled before touching them. Depending where the sore or rash is you may be able to touch around it but you must address it first. Your partner may even be oblivious to their condition and hopefully will be grateful that you are communicating. If it is too uninviting, then you have to go with how you feel and pass on the touching. I have a friend who went to bed with a woman who had a pimply butt. This bothered him and he said that he was unable to have his full attention on her. This is obviously not the same as an unknown rash or disease. Noticing the pimples is one thing, but to dwell on them is pointless. You do not have to communicate about something like that unless it is your close friend whom you know would want to be informed. Just put your attention and focus back on the pleasure. It is like in meditation, your mind will wander but you can just notice that and focus back on your breathing or whatever it is that you are meditating on. And in our case just put your attention back on the feelings of pleasure.

If it is a herpes blister, you of course do not want to rub directly on the affected area or even in the near vicinity. If it is far enough away from the clitoris or penis then we feel that it is safe to pleasure those areas if everyone is on board with it. You can use latex gloves if you have any doubts and definitely wash your hands with soap and water when finished making sure not to touch your own skin before doing so.

Now that we have gotten that out of the way, it is time to touch your partner. As we remind you in the communication section it is helpful to let your partner know ahead of time what you are up to. If you are not familiar with the person you are going to pleasure, ask them about their preferences. If they are unsure about those then ask them simple questions while touching them that they can answer with either a yes or a no. Simple questions such as "More pressure?" "Less pressure" "Faster?" "Slower?" "More to the Left?" Use small incremental changes and keep asking if they answered yes the first time till you find the exact way they like it. Use questions that either yes or no will be an okay answer and will not cause any emotional disturbances. Those are called winning questions. Questions like "Does this feel good?" or "Do you like this?" are poor questions. Emotions might get involved. That is because a person may not want to hurt your feelings and will therefore respond falsely. They also might answer truthfully and say no to those questions. Then you might feel the negativity, and this also could lead to trouble.

Touché'

I like to have the clitoris be the focal point and pretty much touch everywhere else on a woman's body that I am going to touch before zeroing in on it. The same can be done to men using their penis as the focal area. This causes a state of arousal as your partner will feel anticipation and desire to have that erogenous focal point be touched, too. You can start as far away as you like, for example, feet, hands and head—and then work your way towards their genitals. You also do not have to begin so far away and touch wherever you feel like touching like thighs, stomach or breasts to commence. In some scenarios where she or he is so desirous and aroused that you can't resist it, you can start directly on her clitoris or on his penis.

You can also play with energy around your partner's body. Without touching them put your hand close to their skin and see if you or they can detect any sensation. The genitals and other erogenous zones that consist of erectile tissue such as the anus, facial lips, nipples (they erect by a muscle and are not considered actual erectile tissue), ears are probably going to be the most sensitive to this.

Often, I will initiate touch by using my hands, the fingers and even the back of my hand, inner wrist as well as my forearm and even upper arm to lightly touch my partner's thighs after announcing my intentions first. Light, fairly quick stimulation is generally tumescent and the goal is to tumesce her so that might be the usual pressure to start. It also can feel good to start slowly and deliberately so you have to go on a case-by-case scenario and do what feels best to you each time. It is good idea to get into a comfortable position so that you and they can be in a relaxed state and can easily touch them without getting tired or cramped. This is especially true when you get to their genitals so that you can really focus and not be distracted by your own cramped or achy body.

Sometimes your partner will be out of her body and too tumesced already. In that case you could use firm, more deliberate pressure without much movement, just some solid pressure to bring her back into her body so that she will be able to feel what you are doing. This steady pressure can be anywhere on her body that feels right to you such as her upper chest, forehead, abdomen or even thighs and feet. Sometimes just cupping your hand over their whole vulva and firmly pressing will do the trick. The same firm pressure can be used to bring a man back into his body to feel your touch when he is too hyper-excited. It is mostly the intention that you use when touching someone whether the stroke brings him or her up or down. The same stroke with a different intention will cause different results.

You can touch and play around with your partner's non-genitals for as long as you and they are enjoying it. The amount of time also depends on how much time you both have available. The goal is not to give them a massage although that can be fun too. A massage, especially using a lot of pressure, would generally bring them down. The purpose of touching them without involving their genitals, besides just enjoying the sensation of the moment, is to tease them and play with them so that they become aroused and where their genitals will be especially desirous of your touch. You can approach their genitals and then back off. You may brush the pubic hair gently in a flirtatious fashion so that they will feel your attention and intention. Consider your hands and fingers and whatever part of you that you touch your partner with to be sex organs that thoroughly enjoys whatever they are touching. Communicate your delight verbally so that your partner won't feel like they owe you and also to feel more yourself. As we wrote in the communication section, the more you can acknowledge the pleasure you are feeling will also make it easier for them to acknowledge the pleasure that they are feeling, which will help escalate the fun.

Touching a Woman

Let's say now you are ready to focus in further and onto the genitals. Keep the clitoris as the focal point so avoid touching it until she is practically begging you to. I like to play around the area with different pressure and touches before I put any lubricant on. I also like to look at her pussy and see visually how she is responding to my stimulation. Even with my regular partner, Vera, I enjoy the visual experience and notice where she is in her state of arousal with my hands and with my eyes. I like to be playful, so I don't have a specific checklist that I go through but rather do whatever I feel like doing.

Heat Check

The touches are deliberate and some of the things I might do but not all in the same session are:

Putting my hand above the skin to notice any sensation.

Checking the heat that is being generated by her pussy with my hand close to it but not touching. You can place your hand elsewhere above her chest or throat area and see if the heat is being trapped there still without direct skin contact. If it is hotter elsewhere just remind her to bring the energy down to her pussy. You will be surprised at how much the heat can shift. When a person is afraid or nervous a lot of the heat as well as the sensation gets trapped around their throat area. When you play around with this method, the person who is receiving your attention will understand that you are really focused on them if you are reporting to them what they are actually feeling and where. When you tell them to bring the heat down to their pussy they will naturally do so. It is part of the taking control by noticing and enables a person to surrender to you.

Opening the Labia

You may then open her inner labia to get a good view of her pussy. You can use one hand on each side placed on her outer lips or labia majora, with as many fingers as you feel like using that are most enjoyable to you. You will be astonished by how much pressure you will be able to use with most women. That is true for some parts of her body. Generally, when stroking a woman on her clitoris or her nipples she will prefer it on the lighter side but not always and not everyone. It is usually a good idea to start with gentle pressure, then ask if she would care for more pressure and see what the limits might be and what the favored pressure is.

You can also use a single hand to spread the inner labia or a couple of fingers from each hand. I sometimes like to use my index and middle finger of my right hand and place them down so that they are touching one another in the middle of the labia and then spreading them apart slowly and deliberately, taking the inner or labia minora with them on either side to open it up to the light of day. It is just something you can play around with. Inform and report to her what you notice; such as how pink the coloration or any signs of orgasm such as engorgement, lubrication or contractions.

Some women will immediately start contracting from the spreading open of their labia and all the attention focused there. Some women will be noticeably wet from the anticipation. Another thing that I like to do sometimes is just to blow a little puff of air on the clitoral area. You don't have to be the big bad wolf that wants to blow the house down, just enough of a puff to get her attention. You can do this before or after you open her labia. If you notice any contractions, you can report what you see to your partner.

Visualizing the Clitoris

The clitoris is often buried under a hood and requires some pulling or tugging around the area, usually from above to pull back this hood or curtain. A technique that I sometimes use to get a better visualization of her pussy and her clitoris is where I press just above her clitoris on her pelvic area with my palm to expose the clitoris to the air and light from under its hood. You can place your hand perpendicular or parallel to her body, whatever you feel more adept at. Also use incremental pressure to determine what she prefers. You can also pull up with a finger or two above the clitoris to expose it from under the hood. You can even use two hands placed slightly above her clitoris on the lower abdomen to expose the clitoris using as many fingers as you like.

We recommend some type of pulling or tugging to expose the clitoris and again to notice and report what you notice such as coloration, engorgement, or contractions. Make sure you are not pulling any pubic hair by accident. You may be surprised how far you can pull without hurting your partner if done confidently. You can even try the puffing technique when pulling the hood back.

Playing with Her Pubic Hair

You may play with her pubic hair by gently and purposefully brushing it away from her labia minora and away from her clitoris and clitoral hood. You can lightly touch just the ends of her hairs in a deliberate fashion. Enjoy your hand as you do so. You can even tug on a bunch of hair at the same time doing it deliberately if that is something that she has told you that she likes, again using incremental pressure. Not every woman will like this, so don't just think you know more than she does. Ask if she would like to experiment with different pressures and always begin gently and proceed incrementally. Once you have trained with each other you will be more familiar with your partner's preferences. You can also go to the other extreme and barely touch her pubic hair with your hand, back of your hand, your knuckles or with your fingertips. It may be ticklish to some women so try it out consciously and cautiously. See how lightly you can touch her where she can still sense your touch, even moving your hand off and away all together using the same motion as if you were in contact. The hair or the pubic hair in this case is an extension of a person's epidermis and there are a lot of nerve endings in that area. We have noticed a lot of women more so now than ever who shave down there. They could be missing out on some of the fun by having their pubic hair removed but it does make it easier to navigate and visualize this field of dreams. Unless the pubic hair is so thick, bushy and wild we recommend to our students to stop shaving it.

Checking the Pressure

I may put a knuckle or two or three or even my whole fist upon her introitus just inside her inner labia and use increasing pressure to see if this feels good to her. Again, you may be surprised by how much pressure she is able to enjoy. Some women will get off just from this firm pressure while some are less sensitive in this area. You can try using continual pressure or pressing for a second or so, releasing and repeating the pressure again for a number of intervals. You can check out this kind of pressure on her perineum too. Another stroke that

I like to use with my knuckles is to line them up lengthwise so that only the tip of the knuckles touches and to lightly touch between the labia or on the labia or even just on the pubic hair or a combination of all three. You can touch without lubricant on plus after you apply the lubricant on the inner labia you can check out how it feels to slide the knuckles up and down on them. The back of the hand and the knuckles are surprisingly sensitive.

I also have found it quite stimulating for some women to just put one knuckle, usually my left hand index one, firmly yet gently inside the labia pressed up against the introitus similar to the stroke above and leaving it in this position without moving it. This allows the woman to feel me without stroking yet and feel my presence and attention upon her. She can feel safe and the sensation actually can build without my doing anything but being present. I can feel her contractions and pulsations and report any of these orgasmic signs to her.

Hot Dog

I sometimes will put one finger usually my index or middle finger like a hot dog between a bun right on her introitus between her labia and use different pressures to see if she likes that and what pressures she prefers. I am using my whole length of finger where the pad of the finger is facing down and flat. You can also move your whole finger slightly in either direction like a roller, clockwise and counterclockwise to cause a response. You can also place your thumb between the labia on the introitus for a thumb-hot dog or knockwurst stroke. Sometimes, especially with younger women, they will be quite wet and your finger will slide about easily. If it is too dry you many want to wait until you have applied some lubricant to roll around.

You can put a finger flat against her perineum to stimulate that. Just leave it there and communicate what you are doing. You can ask her to feel you. Notice any female lubrication, coloration or contractions and report anything you notice. Imagine your finger as a sex organ and see how much pleasure it can feel. You can also use a couple of fingers or your thumb. You can play with the extremes of pressure.

Find out the lightest stroke that she can feel and the most pleasurable pressure and the maximum pressure she would want you to use.

Squeezing and Poking

Although these words don't sound too sensual, they can be a fun addition. Something that it seems that a lot of women enjoy is to squeeze their clitoris through the hood between the pads of your thumb and index finger. Apply incremental pressures to determine what her preferences are. You can do what I call the yo-yo stroke where I squeeze the clitoris through the hood in such a way that you create kind of a wave like motion, which has the clitoris go up and down like a yo-yo of course. It is kind of like a milking stroke. You can feel the shaft of the clitoris between your fingers. The clitoral head under the hood seems to go into her body and then pops back up between your finger and thumb. You can peak her with this simple stroke. Notice any signs of orgasm and describe what you are doing and what you are noticing. If it does not seem to work exactly like a yo-yo that is okay; at least enjoy whatever sensations you are feeling. By communicating with your partner and having her report to you how it feels to her you can experiment safely and enjoyably. Genital exploration can be an awe-inspiring adventure.

You may also put the clitoris, that is the hooded head and the shaft of the clitoris between the sides of your index and middle finger of one hand and apply different squeezing pressures and rhythms. Use as much length of your fingers that feels right. You can include the labia between your fingers along with the hood at the same time. Besides squeezing in and out you can pull and push the area between your fingers in an up and down motion. The pressure can vary from a fairly strong grip between your fingers where there is no frictional movement to a gentle up and down gliding stroke on the outside of the inner labia and against the hood on both sides at the top of the stroke. You can get a good grip on the entire clitoris with this stroke and when squeezing and stroking here you can feel the engorgement and the growing contractions. Do whatever feels right at the time. You may tug on one side or the other. The above and below research investigations are not meant necessarily to copy verbatim but to generate some fun ideas of your own. All these are some ideas that I've used that you can employ to create your own genital exploratory practice.

You can poke the clitoris through the hood on both the upper left and upper right sides with your one finger. Notice that I have not directly touched her on her clitoral head yet but have been touching it through the hood or on the shaft.

You can explore the lower parts of her clitoris as well coming from below with you fingertip and pressing gently at first on the bottom of the clitoris on the right, left or middle part of it. See if you can feel the clitoral shaft. Feel what you are doing and experiment with different pressures and amount of time pressing and when to release the pressure. We will give you some more information about this area when we describe the lubricating of the pussy.

I may do a couple of the above-mentioned touches at the same time like knuckle pressure and exposing the clitoris or hot dog and poking. I also at times like to surround the clitoris from as many sides at once as I can. I may press the clitoris from underneath with a knuckle or a finger. I can then squeeze the clitoris through the hood with my other hand between two fingers. I can push my hands closer and closer together trapping the clitoris between them from all sides at once so that she knows that it is trapped. I purposefully still have not touched her directly on the flesh of her clitoris or used any deep insertion, but she knows that I have got her where she wants it. I can then allow her to feel this experience of being surrounded, as long as it feels good. I will notice any signs of orgasm such as engorgement, color change or contractions while I am playing around and inform my partner what I notice. I also like to get her to acknowledge any good sensations that she feels.

Doing Guys

Before we get directly on the clitoris, I am going to peak you by changing the subject gender. The best way to touch a man pleasurably is the same as in touching a woman, which is to do it so it feels good to you. You don't have to really do anything spectacular if you are enjoying what you are doing. The harder you work at it the less fun it will be for the both of you. Guys are very visual in general and also respond quickly to turn-on and to pussy suggestions. Just the sight of a woman's naked body generally turns on heterosexual men, especially when she is feeling it. Different males will have different specific female body parts and areas, which turn them on the most. A woman's naked legs turn me on and many other guys. Other men are breast fixated; some are ass oriented. The sight of her pussy is excitable to most hetero males. Even though I really like women's legs, a shoulder, her toned arm, her butt, her pussy can all turn me on. So being a sexy woman you can use whatever part of your body that you like about yourself and that turns you on to arouse your partner. It is helpful to know what his specific turn-ons are and to exploit those when doing him.

Sometimes when Vera is putting sexual attention on my body, I like it when she sits or lies next to me so that I can see her sexy legs. She can flex her calves or show me her inner thigh and I am already in the beginnings of orgasm before she has touched me. I like it when she uses simple fantasy for example: "I am going to pin you down with my strong thighs and then finish you off with my calves." Just writing those words turns me on. I can imagine how much turn on I could feel if there was some real pussy intention behind those words. Just talking about a sexy part of her body and what she can do with it is enough to arouse most guys. Like in the ZZ Top song, "She's got legs and she knows how to use them."

It is helpful to feel your pussy as much as you can when pleasuring a man. It makes it more fun for you and for him. I don't mean that you should be necessarily touching yourself but just having some attention there.

We recommend that it usually is a good idea if the woman is gratified first before she begins to pleasure her partner. It is probably better if she's relaxed and ended on a high level and did not come down too far or go over the edge in a tensed state. Then when she is pleasuring the man, she won't feel needy or be coming from scarcity, but will still have desire. She also will have more sensation in her pussy and it will be easier for her to feel her sensuality as she pleasures him. We know a number of women who if they are going to be only doing the man and not letting him gratify her first will primp before the date and self-pleasure themselves so they will be in a more pleasure giving state.

Then when you do start to touch him take it slow and deliberate, perhaps not quite as deliberate and quite as slow with most men as in doing a woman, but you get the idea. Just like in doing a woman have his penis be the focal point and touch everywhere else but that. Use whatever part of your body that you like on whatever part of his body that you feel like touching; you can use the back of your arms, your fingers, your fingernails, the hair on your head, your feet and more, and remember to touch for your own pleasure. It can be fun to put heavier pressure on his lower abdomen or lighter strokes on his upper thighs. Some men like their nipples fondled and as I've stated I have a connection with my facial lips, so I like them played with. Ask him if there is any part of his body that he enjoys having touched and what kind of pressure he likes on that area. Determine if your partner has any connections that he has developed or that are natural. Exploit those and whatever you desire to touch. Just resting your hand almost anywhere on his body and feeling your pussy will be arousing to him. The wild fast jack rabbit motion can be used at some appropriate times, yet the slow deliberate and sensual non-movement can be more provocative. And it is a lot easier.

Lubrication

I am going to peak you some more at this point by discussing the use of lubrication on the genitals. In some ways it is not a little peak but a heightening of the sensual act. It can even be the most fun part of the whole experience. I love when someone puts the lubricant on me with style and feeling. I love applying the lubricant to women when they are ready for it and to myself when I am self-pleasuring. Sometimes all

I will do is apply the lubricant sensually to myself, which could take a few minutes and then wiping it off with a towel. It can be that much fun. It is sheer joy.

Remember to touch for your own pleasure. It has to feel wonderful to your fingers as you do it. I will discuss a number of ways we recommend applying the lubrication to a penis and several ways I like to apply it to a woman's genitals. We gave you a description in the self-pleasuring section already and by learning how to do it to yourself you can teach your partner to do it to you similarly. Putting on the lubricant can be a real thrill for either a man or a woman if done in the spirit of sensual play. Experiment with different lubricants and enjoy the application. You can use one finger or your whole hand.

Lubricating a Penis

There are all kinds of ways to lubricate a male. One way that feels especially good is doing it slowly and deliberately, a little area at a time saving his most sensitive area just below the head of his penis on the ventral side for last. You can also lubricate his penis quickly just taking a big blob of lubricant and coating his penis all at once or any speed between those two. It is nice if he is hard and ready when you apply the lubricant but often it may not be engorged yet. Do not fret about that. It still feels good to him to pleasurably have his member played with in any condition. The more you put your attention on the fun and the less on the productivity and the success the better it will feel. The application of the lubricant will often be the stimulus that causes further engorgement.

I usually like the slow sensual way the best. Be sure that you are comfortable and relaxed. Take a little lubricant on your index finger and put a little bit on the lower part of his penis, which is usually less sensitive than the area near the corona or head. Continue to spread some lubricant on the back or dorsal side of his lower part of his penis and slowly spread it around that area so that it is a thin coat. Then you can take some more lubricant and do the same for the ventral or underneath side of his penis and the side edges too. Then you can lube up the top portion of the back or dorsal side and go from there and apply slowly and deliberately around the head of the penis. So now the only area that is not lubricated is the top ventral side just below the corona or area right under the head. This area is also called the apex. Then slowly make sure that you coat everything but that most sensitive area. Then if he has a circumcised penis take a small blob of lubricant and lightly put it on the apex doing so without at first directly touching your finger against the skin of his penis. Just have the lubricant touching and lightly spread that on. Eventually touch it gently with your finger. Feel his response as you touch his most sensitive spot. If he is not circumcised, you will have to push back that extra skin to get to his apex. You can play for a while on this sensitive are or you can go back and take one finger and lightly touch the penis all over again to make sure that the whole penis is coated with lubricant. Make sure to enjoy your finger as you touch him.

Sometimes it can be fun to take a big glob of lubricant on your hand and then gently but firmly grab his penis and glide your hand slowly around to make sure that the lubricant is spread all over it. You can also just hold the member and lightly squeeze it and release it and squeeze it and release it as many times as it feels good. You can keep doing the squeeze part for as long or as short as you like. It does not have to be totally rhythmical. It should feel good to the hand and to the penis.

Being that I have leg fantasies, I have taught Vera to sometimes apply the lubricant with her finger pretending to be a leg, where the knuckle is her knee, the tip of the finger mimics her foot while the lower section of her finger simulates her thigh and the area between the joint and the fingertip feigns to be her calf. She can apply the lube this way using a different part of her leg I mean finger for different areas of my penis. She can then hold my penis between her bent finger, as if she had me inside her knee joint, verbally teasing my imagination as she does so.

Lubricating a Pussy

I like to tease a woman first without touching her clitoris and the same goes for when I put the lubricant on. I want her to feel as much as possible each step in the process and don't want to apply the lubricant too soon or too late. I want to feel that she is primed and ready for the slippery yummy sensation of the application of the slick and smooth feeling on her pussy when the lubricant is being applied.

Being that Vera is close to eighty years old, it is extra necessary to lubricate her genitals and women of her age before any serious rubbing and stroking. Younger women will be less dry and there is a good chance that they will be quite wet and self-lubricated at this point anyway. It still can be a lot of fun to apply the lubricant perhaps in a smaller amount on the already wet inner labia and introitus. We recommend that you do not apply any lubricant on the outer labia as we usually don't stroke there and it will just make things too greasy. Additionally, it is best not to use any lubricant on the clitoral hood, as this will make it too slippery for when you want to pull it back at some point away from the clitoris to expose the clitoris.

I like to take a small glob of lubricant and put it on the back of my left hand as a reservoir, as I am right handed and do most of the genital stroking with my right hand and fingers. Being that I apply the lubricant somewhat differently each time I do it I will give you a couple of examples and you can create your own ways too.

I will put a little bit of the lubricant on my middle or index finger. I will then spread apart the inner labia with either just my left hand or with both hands, where I use the bottom or side of my right hand or even my thumb so that my finger with the lubricant is free to move around the genitals. Sometimes I like to spread the lubricant and separate the labia with my right hand only and use my left hand to pull back her hood and kind of stretch her entire vulva. This stretching also places the clitoris further away from her labia so that you won't accidentally bump into it. This stretching also usually feels good to her. I will place the palm of my left hand perpendicularly and right above her clitoris and press against this area and pull upwards to cause this elongation.

Whatever technique I am using, I will slowly and surely with verbal communication as to what I am doing place the finger with the lubrication against the perineum. You can start anywhere on her genitals that you like, preferably saving her clitoral head for last. I can see the opened pussy and report how beautiful she is. I will go gently at first without much movement and then use a little more pressure and a little movement to feel the spread of the lubricant and the response to my touch. If it feels good, I can continue to play in this area, using little longer strokes if that feels right for as long as it demonstrates pleasure. I can also play with diverse pressures and the speeds of the little strokes here. Sometimes I will put some lubricant on the tip of my finger and apply the lubricant without spreading the labia first. I slowly press my finger inside the labia and on the introitus. The labia will then open on their own. I then continue as before. At some point it will be right to move away from this area. It could be a few seconds or up to a few minutes.

I will then remove my finger and put some more lubricant on the tip of my middle or index finger. I will then as I did before with communication and spreading of the labia apply the lubricant to the inside of one of the labia; let's say the right side first. I still might be using my second hand to stretch the vulva. Lightly but deliberately, I will slowly coat the entire right labia from the perineum to near the clitoris. I may then do some light slow stroking up and down that labia. I can again play with different speeds and diverse pressures; from light slow ones to firmer slow stokes, from long quick light strokes to short quick ones on a specific area of the labia. The upper part of the labia that is nearest the clitoris is often very sensitive and light little quick strokes here can be very stimulating and pleasurable to her.

The left labia is probably getting jealous so I communicate to my partner that I am going to move my finger to the left side and then remove it and put a little more lubricant on my finger tip. I then proceed to play with the left labia in a similar fashion as I did the right one making sure that the entire introitus or vaginal opening is coated and primed too. I can spend as much time as it is fun with the labia. Once both sides are coated and neither of them are no longer jealous, I can go back and forth between the two sides with whatever strokes feel appropriate, getting as close to the clitoris as I dare. I will sometimes do a bunch of short light quick strokes on the upper labia of one side and then move to the other side and do some short quick strokes there and go back and forth between these two areas. The amount of strokes can vary so you can do one or two or a dozen or thirty or whatever feels good to you. It helps if the woman has a connection between the labia and her clitoris. Vera can really get off well with just the stroking of her labia especially the area close to the clitoris. We have met some women who were more sensitive on this part of their genitals than even their clitoris. We have also had students with all kinds of labial sizes. Some were large and some were hardly visible. You will have to notice and accommodate whatever you are presented with and enjoy that. There is no normal in this context.

I also like to go up and down the introitus where I approach the clitoris slowly from below and then reverse as if Sisyphus rolling the rock first up the hill and then all the way back down to her perineum. Finally, after some teasing, I will gain enough momentum upwards and make it all the way to the bottom of the clitoris and use some pressure without any stroking movement against it. Many women will respond with fairly strong contractions at this point. We called it the Michael Douglas stroke because he, as well as a lot of other actors, seem to fuck in movies standing up, pressing the woman against a wall. It is that pressure against a wall that we were simulating. It is important to feel the firm and perhaps spongy bottom of the clitoris here and to push it back where it feels like it is against a wall. Also be aware of how much pleasure is being felt. Only do it if it is fun for her. Notice that we have still not touched the head of the clitoris. By continuing to stretch her vulva with your second hand you will have more control over this stroke.

Another example of pussy lubrication is that sometimes I will just coat my entire middle finger with lubricant and place it between her labia like in the previously mentioned hot dog stroke and move it around so that it coats the entire labia. This can be done quickly or slowly depending on what you are feeling in response. Once the tissue is coated with lubricant you can continue to roll your finger in between the labia or change to using your fingertip and start stroking the introitus or labia as I described above.

A third example is to take a large glob of the lubricant on your index and middle fingertips and start applying at the perineum and bringing your fingers slowly up the middle of the introitus or outer part of the vagina, making sure to cover the areas of the labia as you travel up towards the clitoris. This way each finger can play with its own labia at the same time and there will be no unnecessary jealousy. Stop short of the clitoris and clitoral hood. Once the genital tissue is all lubricated you can continue to play with those two fingers up and down and around on the lubricated area or switch to one finger if that feels better.

Another way that I like to apply the lubricant on occasion is to use the knuckle of my middle finger. It seems easier for me to use my left hand as I pull back on the hood and spread the labia with my right hand. You can also use the index finger's knuckle or both knuckles at the same time. I put some lubricant on it and bend my hand almost into a fist. Then with the knuckle sticking out from the rest of the fist I gently rub it along the inside of the labia starting at the perineum and applying it against the introitus. It feels smooth as the knuckle glides along. You can shift it against either labia and move it up and down or side to side or around or whatever feels like it would be the most pleasurable. You can turn your hand around about 90 degrees so that all the knuckles are lined up along the introitus and slickly touch the coated surface. You can then switch to your finger pad or whole finger to play some more.

7
Giving Pleasure —Touchdown

In this chapter you will find out what to do when you finally get your hands on your partner's most sensitive areas. I will start with the man's genitals. Then I will provide a detailed account of how to pleasure a woman. Even though there is quite a bit of difference, there are also a lot of similarities between males and females. Whichever gender you may be or whichever one you may prefer you will do well to read all of the descriptions that follow.

Holding and Embracing the Penis

We have given you a bunch of information already on how to touch a penis in this book and elsewhere. The most important aspect in touching a penis manually is to enjoy what you are doing. Touch it like you are touching a silky outfit or soft fur; that is to make your hand feel pleasure. Get in a comfortable position and take a break whenever you feel like changing your position. You are not required to squirt him or massage him, just to feel pleasure and he will respond to that.

The following are some of the ways that are enjoyable to begin but you can do whatever feels good. You have already lubricated him, and he will probably be somewhat engorged from that. If he is not engorged, you and he can still enjoy your touching it. Start slowly and hold his penis in your hand. Feel the penis, feel how it throbs and its texture. Feel how it engorges. Notice his responses and report to him what you notice. Get your whole hand around it; still not moving your hand just feeling it. Don't just grab it but take it lovingly into your hand. It is kind of like a handshake, firmly but not too firm.

After just feeling it for a while, you can gently squeeze it rhythmically, slowly, tenderly at first and then adding on more pressure gradually with communication. (Note: Do not use too much pressure as this could irritate the urethra.) You can hold the penis for as long as you both enjoy the pressure, staying in communication. When you are between squeezes, keep feeling his penis, too. You may also tug or pull on his member as you are holding it fast in your hand. These can also vary from little tugs to larger pulls. You can also move his penis around in small and then larger circles if he likes that. You can move it from side to side or up and down. You are still not stroking his penis, just taking control of it to check out what it is capable of. We sometimes jokingly compare this to checking out the gears of a stick shift on a manual transmission car. You can go back to your automatic if it is too much work. It is always best to start slowly and gradually use more pressure. Perhaps you did similar touches without lubricant. Communicate with your partner about what feels best.

Stroking the Penis

When stroking a woman, we usually recommend short strokes but with a guy the long strokes all the way up and all the way down his shaft without losing contact at any point are advised. Use all of your hand with as much surface area in contact at all times. When you get toward the top of the penis, it usually is best to lighten up, as that is the most sensitive area for most men. Repeat the same stroke rhythmically so that the sensation builds.

Every man will respond differently when being stroked. The same guy may even respond differently on different occasions. Some guys will be sensitive and get close to ejaculation after a few strokes. Other guys will take many minutes. This is where good communication will inform you where he is. If you are experienced, you will be able to notice just when to peak him similarly as with doing a woman. The disparity is that if you go one stroke too many, he may ejaculate and his party will be over for the time being.

Men who have trained to have an extended massive orgasm will be able to tell you when to stop before they ejaculate. They may be in an orgasmic state with contractions and full engorgement rather quickly. They can sustain the orgasm and have the intensity increase with every peak. They might seep or leak ejaculate, but they won't squirt if you are conscious of their arousal and peak them at the right time.

Once you get a man almost to ejaculation and have peaked him you will notice that the next strokes that you do will bring him up probably very quickly with very few strokes necessary. The longer you wait between peaks will mean that he has gone down further, and it will take longer to bring him back up again. You can tease him with words using his favorite fantasies and your turned-on body to keep him on edge.

You can check out all kinds of strokes on the various peaks that you give him. You can rub his penis with just one finger or just your thumb along the urethra on the ventral side. You can go all the way up and down his shaft or just stay in a small zone for example the most sensitive area under his corona on the underneath or ventral side of his penis. You can use a twisting motion with your whole hand like on a spiral staircase. You can keep your hand in one vertical area of his shaft and move your hand horizontally back and forth. You can check out different angles for your hand depending on where you are located in relation to your partner.

You can use your thumb or your fingertips along his urethra or vary it as with the spiral motion. You can use a straight hand touching his penis with the palm of your hand or with your finger or fingers. By straight I mean that it is an open hand and not grabbing the penis. You can slide your hand up and down or in circles; whatever feels good to you to do. You can push his penis back toward his belly so that his ventral or underneath side is now facing up and you have access to this most sensitive side with your open hand. You can then stroke him deliberately and sensually with your open hand in this vulnerable yet tantalizing position.

Two Hands on Male Genitals

We are going to expand on some of the information that we gave you in the self-pleasuring chapter. One way that you can use both hands is where you can go up and down with two hands on the shaft at the same time, keeping both in contact at all times. One hand is above the other. You can also take both hands at once and kind of make a basket or pouch with your hands and use them together to hold his penis or rub up and down his shaft as you see fit. You will really have his penis surrounded. You can also do the open-handed technique we just described above but with both hands at once.

You can also stroke with one hand along the shaft from the base to the head of his penis bringing this hand up and over the head of his penis. Then remove your hand by letting go of his penis while at the same time your other hand is starting to stroke upwards from the base. When you have removed your first hand off the top put that hand back to its starting position at the base of his penis and start stroking it upward. Your second hand moves upward along the shaft and over the head of his penis and so on and on. This way all the strokes are starting from the base and go up the pole. There is always one hand at least in contact with his penis. You can do these with a simple up motion or a spiraling one. Remember to notice his state of arousal as this can be quite tantalizing to a man. You do not want him to ejaculate unless you are both ready to finish the cycle. You can check out doing it similarly but in a downward stroke fashion to see how those compare with the upward strokes.

You can also use your second hand to cup his testicles while you are stroking his penis with your primary hand. You can fondle or even pull out on his testicles at the same time you are stroking his penis. One way of pulling on them is to put a couple of fingers around the area between his penis and testes and pulling down with those fingers. You still have a few fingers left to support or caress his testicles as you control his scrotum with your two fingers. You can lightly touch them or massage them more firmly depending on what he prefers. You may additionally pull on his testicles by taking them in your full hand surrounding them. Experiment and be playful. Ask him questions to find out what he enjoys and what he would like.

You can play with the engorged area under the testicles or by his perineum, which is the external zone between them and his anus. You can also feel what we call his hidden cock in this area. It is just an extension of his penis that goes into his body and is not externally visible. It will be engorged just like the rest of his penis. You can stroke this area in a similar pattern and rhythm that you are using on his visible penis or just hold your hand or finger or even your fist there to provide some pressure. The prostate gland is also in this area but buried further inside his body behind the hidden cock toward the testicles. It can feel enjoyable to be massaged externally but remotely. Communicate to find out the pressure he prefers. You can even peak a man when he is about to ejaculate by pressing firmly on this area but as my urologist said this can be harmful to some men. By pressing on this area, you can control the emission of ejaculate either encouraging or stopping its flow. By keeping one hand on his penis and the other under his testicles near his prostate and alternating where and when you are stroking him, you can extend his orgasm for as long as it is fun. You can also peak a guy who is about to ejaculate by squeezing the head of his penis firmly although this again could be harmful to some men. I prefer to be peaked a little sooner by just stopping all motion with no firm pressure or squeezing but some guys might like it this way.

I like my pelvic area pressed firmly in a rhythm when I feel aroused in synch with the stroking of my penis. One can do this with the palm of your hand or with fingers. You can check out what feels best to your partner. You can play with his anal area if you and he are so inclined. Use lubricant and always begin gently on the outside of his anus till you know your partner's limits and yours. Some men like the insertion and you can even massage his prostate from inside his anus. I am too squeamish to appreciate too much insertion, but your guy might like it.

As always proceed gradually and gently at first. Play with a lot of lubricant on the outside of his anus first. When he is relaxed and receptive you can enter gently with one of your fingers, also well lubricated. You can use a fitted latex glove or even a latex finger. It is best to make sure you wash well before and after. The prostate is located about two inches deep into his rectum. Use the pad of your finger to gently press and massage this walnut sized gland. If he is lying on his back, press upwards toward the front of his body with your inserted finger. You cannot directly touch it as the rectal wall separates it from the rectum, but you will be able to find it fairly easily. It will feel spongy. Do not press too strongly as it has a lot of nerve receptors and blood vessels that could bruise. Find out what pressure feels best to your partner. It is better to continue stimulating his penis with one hand as you progress. By pressing on his prostate when he is about to ejaculate you can stop his ejaculation like we discussed earlier. You can stop and restart stroking his penis when you peak him like this to extend his orgasm.

You can do whatever pleasurable things come into your mind or whatever he asks for that seems like fun to you. Communicate and find out if that is something he might enjoy.

Ejaculation

A lot of men like to have an ejaculation to end their cycle of pleasure. Some people enjoy finishing a man off like that and sometimes they may have had enough before he has gotten to that point. Either way is okay. If your partner wants to ejaculate and you are not up for that he can always finish himself off. It is probably a good idea to communicate your preferences up front before beginning so that no one feels betrayed at the end.

If you do take him through the ejaculatory phase, keep the communication lines open. You have peaked him a number of times and this time you want to take him all the way home. You could have squirted him a number of times earlier but you have been practicing peaking and stopped right before he did. He may have had a secondary erection that is the sure tell sign of an impending ejaculation. The head of his penis gets even more engorged and a deeper purple in color. When you are ready to squirt him use your intention in doing so. Some men like it when you speed it up some to take him over. Find out what your partner likes.

You can even tell him "Get ready! I am going to squirt you now," or "I'm going to take you all the way," or something to that effect. You can even peak him a couple of times by stopping and then starting again, communicating how you just baited him but "this time for sure." When you do take him all the way be sure to keep stroking as he ejaculates. Also remember to keep feeling your hand and enjoy this new sensation, as some people go a little spacy when their partners start squirting. As he first begins to squirt you can repeat the same strokes that got him to this point. Usually after a very little while, it is a good idea to lighten your stroke and slow down gradually to keep the ejaculation going as long as possible. Communicate with your partner to find out what he likes and experiment with variations too.

Ejaculation is optional. Once a man learns how to feel an extended massive orgasm he may no longer feel the need to ejaculate just like a woman who has been trained to relax and feel every stroke to its utmost. I don't squirt every time but once in a while I like to experience the big finale. Only rub on his penis as long as you are enjoying it. The goal is always pleasure and fun. If it is no longer enjoyable stop doing it or at least take a break. Some guys just take a long time and others just a couple of strokes. Have it be more fun with some additional intention and he might just go for it too. If you are getting pissed at him for taking so long it definitely is time for a break and some communication. Sometimes if a man has consumed too much alcohol, he may have a "whiskey hard-on," and may take forever to ejaculate.

On the Clitoris

Once you sense that she is ready for some clitoral stroking and that anymore teasing will be overkill; you can get on her spot and start stroking. There are myriad ways that you can do this, too, and they all involve pulling back on the hood to expose the head of the clitoris to your fingertip and to your vision.

Two Handed Do

This is the standard way of stroking a woman's pussy and is a vital stroke to learn.

Get your non-clitoral stroking hand in position first where your thumb is at the base of her introitus pressing gently but firmly downward without any penetration.

Your four remaining fingers are placed under her buttocks, two under each cheek so that you have a snug yet gentle grip there with no extra space between your hand and her body. This means that your fingers are placed as deeply as you can under her buttocks and still have it feel good to you and to her. Depending on the size of the woman's body and her rear end and the size of your hands this grip may vary to some extent. If she is really large or really small you will have to adjust your hand.

This hand is there for a couple of key reasons. The first is that you can feel the contractions and the strength of them with your thumb precisely placed. The other reason is that it feels good to your partner and it should feel good to you. She can relax into your hand and feel your extra attention. You can also tell whether she is lifting up and tensing or is being relaxed and sunk in snugly against your hand. Sometimes while I am stroking the clitoris after she has been feeling it for some time, I may squeeze her butt cheeks to some extent. I usually do so briefly either to get her attention or to take her up a notch and because it feels good to do so.

Anchoring and Exposing the Clitoris

First put a little bit of lubricant on the tip of your index finger or your middle finger depending on which one you will be using. Then you can expose the clitoris by placing the meaty part of your thumb of your stroking hand firmly against the left side of her hood and pulling in an upward direction toward her abdomen. This is also called anchoring because by keeping your thumb pressed up against the clitoral hood you keep the clitoris from moving around. I am right-handed so I will use that as my stroking hand. If you are left-handed then use your left thumb as an anchor against the upper right side of her hood and your left middle finger or index finger to stroke with.

Some people teach that all doers should use their left hand but that is just based on a myth. Use your hand that is most dexterous. Use the hand that you write with, throw with, or brush your teeth with to stroke the clitoris. It is a two handed do so you will be using both hands in tandem.

I regularly do a meditation that I learned from Frank Kinslow (multiple books from Hay House), where I sit quietly and put my attention on my body. I go through the whole body focused on one area at a time. One only spends a few seconds on each area.

I have noticed that the three areas that are most a-buzz for me are my hands, the bottom of my feet and my facial lips, even more so than my penis. My left hand maybe even slightly more sensitive than my right but that makes it a perfect tool to feel a pussy with. My right hand is more dexterous and agile and better for stroking. This makes for a great combination. Baseball analogy: I put the baseball glove on my left hand and do most of the catching with it. I use my right hand to throw with. If I put my glove on my right hand and threw with my left, I would not be a very good fielder. I could practice it that way and I would surely gain some enhancement, but it seems it would be smarter to do it the way that felt right from the beginning.

Now once you pull back on the hood you should be able to see the head of the clitoris clearly. Sometimes the clitoris is so small, or the hood is so tight or does not move at all, that you still won't be able to see the head of the clitoris but with the majority of women, you will be ready to proceed. Even if the hood does not retract completely you can still get your finger placed in the proper zone. Frequently, once the clitoris is stroked it will engorge more and be more clearly defined and visible.

You should be able to clearly visualize different areas of the clitoris such as an upper or top portion that consists of a left, middle, and right zone. You can also usually clearly make out the bottom side of the clitoral head with its three zones. Most women but not all are most sensitive or have the most sensation on the upper left side of their clitoral head. The location that we are referring to is in respect to the woman's body not where you are situated so it is always the same, like her left hand is always her left hand. Now in some cases a woman may prefer or have more sensation on the upper right or even the lower portion of her clitoris and do not argue with her if she believes this. I have found that even if you are doing the same woman over and over that she may prefer that you stroke her on a different side or area on singular occasions. Once you have begun peaking your partner you can test the different areas yourself. One of the most important factors here is that she knows that you know what you are doing and where you are stroking. Once she gets going and is in an intense orgasmic condition; anywhere you touch on her clitoris will feel fantastic if she knows that you are doing so deliberately.

A friend asked me what to do if you know you are on her spot but she is not experiencing much sensation? First, I would give her a chance to start to feel more by just leaving my finger there without moving or stroking with it. I would tell her what I was doing. If she were still resistant, I would offer to check out other spots and areas on her clitoris to determine if those feel better. I would probably take a break first and communicate some more about what I propose to do. Have fun and enjoy all the challenges placed in the way. If you do so, she will eventually feel good, almost regardless of where you are touching.

Getting on the Spot

Now getting back to getting your finger on the spot. The way that we begin the stroke is to bend and hook the doing finger in such a way that it is rubbing in that small zone of the clitoris with short, repetitive and rhythmical strokes up and down so that it stays in the quadrant that you have decided and agreed to stroke, which is usually the upper left. You are just using the tip of the finger and you are gently stroking the area up and down with short strokes. You can actually feel the crease at the top of the clitoral head at the top of the stroke with your fingertip. Your finger or hand is at slight angle so that you can stroke in that area between one and two o'clock if it is the upper left quadrant that you are stroking. This makes for a very small area of the clitoris that you are stroking. If you can stay in this small area at will, the woman can be sure of your aim and dexterity.

We have noticed that most guys will still use too long a stroke even when you tell them to use a short stroke. The shorter the stroke the better is a good rule to go by.

We have found though that some women who are new to having their clitorises directly touched will prefer a longer stroke and one that even takes the finger away from the clitoris as part of the stroke. This way it is not quite as intense. A lot of guys when they are first learning how to stroke a clitoris will unconsciously use a longer stroke thinking that they are on the clitoris the whole time. This makes for a perfect couple only they won't get very far together like this. It will be difficult to make progress. It is okay to leave the spot but is best to do so deliberately and consciously. Then she will know that you know what you are doing. One way around this is that you can give her a couple short strokes and then tell her you will give her a couple longer ones. That way she will feel your attention and deliberateness and can surrender to you more easily.

A lot of women like it very light especially when you start to touch there and some women who are new to having their clitoris touched are too sensitive to have it stroked at all. We have described this condition in the self-pleasuring chapter. Proceed slowly. It is okay to first rub on the hood or nearby to avoid direct contact. Eventually if she desires to feel more you can get a glob of lubricant and touch her clitoris through the lubricant without touching it directly with your fingertip. You can then try a quick press and release directly on her spot with some lubricant without stroking it. If that feels good, then you can try some more presses without stroking yet. Finally, if she is still up for more try stroking it only one or two strokes at a time very gently. By taking your time and having patience she will open up and allow you to touch it more and more.

Our original teacher was really good at doing but had a very large hand with thick fingers and therefore it was more difficult for him to locate it in a small zone. He was able to overcome this handicap with his strong intention and ability to feel and respond to what his partner was feeling. People seem to allow a person who has extreme well-deserved confidence to take control of their sensual beingness. It is more important than the actual placement of one's fingers. The combination of precision and confidence is even better.

Exposing Clitoris by Other Means

One of my favorite strokes to use instead of anchoring and exposing the clitoris with my thumb is to pull back and press down on the pelvic area right above the clitoris with the palm of my clitoris-doing hand to accomplish this. The palm is parallel to her body so that your fingers can get to the clitoris easily. This placement is different to the one I described earlier as I recommended a perpendicular position for using your second hand to pull back the hood with. This stroke is easier than the thumb anchoring one to learn but is better suited to do after the clitoris is already engorged and more stabilized. Therefore, it still is a good idea to learn how to anchor with your thumb.

When you pull back and expose the clitoris with your palm you can use your index or middle finger to stimulate whatever region of her clitoris that she and you desire. It can also add to the pleasure at times by rhythmically pressing down with your palm at the same time you are stroking with your finger. While your partner may prefer light pressure on her clitoris, she may like some firmer pressure on her lower abdomen. It always is a good idea to ask your partner if they would like more pressure and to gradually add it on. Once you have trained each other then you will know her favorite pressures to use and if she wants you to change that then all they have to do is to ask.

The main function of the palm in this position is to expose the clitoris from under the hood. The trick is to pull back with enough pressure to expose the clitoris but not too much where it will be painful. A variation of this stroke is to expose the clitoris with the other hand on her pelvis. This will of course take your hand away from her buttocks and introitus. Then you can stroke with your regular doing hand with either the thumb anchoring or not. When a person is first learning how to do, it sometimes simplifies things to expose the clitoris in this fashion. If done right, the clitoris will be visually wide-open and available. You won't have to crook and bend your finger as much to get on her spot and this will allow you to keep your strokes light without having to dig under her hood as you would with the thumb doing the uncovering. Once she is fully engorged you can also use the pad of your finger as well as your fingertips in this position.

Clitorises and their hoods vary so much. Remember the snowflake analogy. Some clitorises seem like there is no hood covering them at all and are visible without any pulling back of the hood. Others will be extremely difficult to view no matter how well you pull back the hood. In these cases, you will have to rely on your sense of touch alone. By hooking your finger under the hood and digging under the hood you will be able to feel the clitoris and reach and stroke any area that you choose to. It still is a good idea to learn to use your thumb in the anchoring position, as it will keep the clitoris from moving around which it often tends to do, especially if she is resisting your control.

The size of the clitoris also varies greatly among different women. Some are really large, and the different quadrants are totally visible and available with visible middle quadrants available. Some clitorises are so tiny that there really is no way to differentiate a unique quadrant. The intensity of the pleasure that a woman feels is not related to the size of her clitoris. Additionally, once you start stroking the clitoris it will engorge. It is similar to a penis in that respect. If you find yourself rubbing on a small clitoris don't worry about finding a spot or specific quadrant. Enjoy touching for the pleasure it gives you, as you should be doing anyway. The stroke is the same, that is short and usually on the left side, just that you won't be able to stay in that specific quadrant, as your finger is too big to do that. Be open-minded and explore all areas of her clitoris that you can.

We have met women who had no hood or that their clitoris stuck out naturally without having to pull back the hood at all. It still is a good idea to anchor it with your thumb so that it does not move around on you. Clitorises even well exposed ones can be slippery and tricky. It does make it easier to maneuver your finger on it, but the orgasm will not be any more intense than those with large hoods. The other extreme is where the hood does not move, and you cannot get directly on the clitoris. You can rub through the hood with a normal stroke and that can still feel great to the woman. I also found that there might be a small spot at the bottom of the clitoris kind of where it meets the labia and a little of the clitoris may be exposed here. I was able to directly touch there with one of the women who had this condition. It was where she experienced the most pleasure. It's fun to explore and experiment on whatever feels best. Everyone is built differently, and you will have to study on an individual basis to determine what your partner likes best.

Stroking the Clitoris

Once you have your lubricated fingertip on her spot you can start stroking it if she is ready to go for a ride. Once you know where her favorite spot is and you are on it just use a short up and down stroke, feeling your finger in both directions. Keep repeating the same exact stroke for as long as it is pleasurable to you and as long as she keeps going for her pleasure. As long as the intensity is increasing you can keep stroking with the same stroke. At some point she will not be going up anymore. You would like to take a break and peak her right before this happens. Use the communication skills that we gave you in that chapter.

Each peak should consist of one type of rhythmical stroke. You can peak her by changing the stroke as well as by stopping. So, you can either change the location of the stroke, the pressure or the speed that you are using. You can use a longer stroke too once she knows that you know where her spot is. It is usually a good idea to go back to her spot frequently. I often will use a couple long slow strokes down her introitus or labia and then back up again to bring her down a little before I go back on her spot to give her another peak.

You can also do a stroke where you are on the spot for a few strokes then on the other side of her clitoris, then on the upper middle, and then on the bottom and then back to her spot. This is better done when she is fully engorged and receptive to whatever you throw her way. Even though you are moving your finger around to different areas, it is one basic rhythm that is involved.

I like to have some music playing so that I can use the rhythm of the individual songs to dance or stroke upon her clitoris according to the beat (but you can also make the music in your head if your partner finds it distracting). You can then peak her by just skipping one or two beats and then continue the dance. This is like dipping her if you were really dancing. Sometimes the music will change, and you can go with that change and other times you may want to stroke at your own beat.

As noted before, there are numerous ways to expose her clitoris from under the hood. You can change the way you are exposing it from the thumb technique to your palm pressed above her clitoris. This is another way to peak her by shifting your hand around. Again, once she is fully engorged you can more easily use the pressed palm technique and switch over to your middle finger if you like. Then you can continue with whatever rhythmical stroke you feel like using. The length of the peaks will vary so you have to keep being aware of her orgasmic curve.

Another stroke that you can do is to instead of going up and down with your finger moving about on her clitoris to kind of stay attached to one spot and jiggling your finger so that the clitoris is still moving but your finger is in the same place. It is almost like a vibrator stroke using the pressure she prefers. You can also try circles, either little ones or larger ones. You can go side to side, going left to right and back again. You can try a Morse code kind of stroke where you touch and release and touch and release but doing so in a specific rhythm.

You can make up any type of touch that you can think of. The basic short stroke in the pocket or favorite spot is one you are best to rely on and to go back to when you really want her to take it up to a higher level of intensity.

While you are stroking with your doing hand you are feeling with your second hand. You can just leave your thumb there firmly placed against the base of her introitus or once she gets going in a nice pattern, you can move that thumb up and down and around her introitus to add additional sensation. Its main function remains always to use it as a meter to determine how the orgasm is progressing.

Vaginal Insertion

Here are some insertion techniques that you can add to the sensation produced while stroking the head of the clitoris. Remember the most important part is still the direct stimulation of the clitoris.

At some point of stroking the clitoris, a woman may have desire for some penetration added. Your thumb that is snug on the base of her introitus is viable to be sucked into her vagina. We suggest not forcing anything. With real desire it will just kind of get sucked into her. If it feels right, you can use a little more pressure and play with the thumb pad facing and pressing down going as far down as feels right. There is a "thunk" (feels good) spot at six o'clock inside of her vagina. You can use an up and down or really an in and out motion to stimulate this area going at whatever speed feels right to just leaving it there without much motion. You can also raise the thumb to the twelve o'clock top of her vagina anterior side where the G-spot is located. You can use the nail side of your thumb to play with this area. It is under where her clitoris is. The nail should be short and have no sharp edges. You can also play with the three o'clock and the nine o'clock segments inside of her vagina, as they all are thunk spots. The thumb cannot go as deep as your fingers can.

You can also use two fingers in place of the thumb once you know that she wants some penetration. You can use a come-hither type of stroke with as much pressure as feels right and that she approves of.

You can go as deep into the vagina as you and she desire as long as that feels best. You do not want to go straight down inside her vagina as you might poke her cervix, as this can be uncomfortable, although recently we met a woman who liked her cervix touched. Hopefully she is wet, but if not, make sure that you use proper lubrication. As I related older women are not as wet as younger ones in general. It should feel good to you as well as to her to rub inside at the same time as you stroke outside on the clitoris.

You can do any of the areas or thunk spots inside her vagina with your two fingers that you did with your thumb. You can probably get some good deep strokes going easier than with your thumb. You can add more fingers inside her vagina if she likes that, but two fingers is usually plenty. If it is tight in the beginning, you can even start with one finger and then add a second one if it loosens up. The come-hither motion is a good reliable movement but you can check out any kinds of motion that you both agree on and that feels pleasurable. By massaging and stimulating her vagina this way you may cause more of her female ejaculate to be secreted and excreted.

Some women don't like to be stroked exactly at twelve o'clock high inside the vagina because their urethral canal is located there and it can feel uncomfortable to be stroked directly. Some women do not mind being stroked there so you will have to find out on an individual basis. Go a little to the sides of this zone when stimulating this area to be on the safe side at first; like at eleven and one o'clock. This is where the G-Spot is located. It will feel engorged and bulbous to the touch about an inch and a half to two inches inside and to the anterior of her vagina or about up to your second joint of your finger.

As the G-Spot area engorges the Paraurethral/Skenes glands located in that area can secrete ejaculate that empties into the urethra and if a woman pushes out she can experience a female ejaculate if aroused. It is not something that we teach our students, as it can take away from their being present minded to becoming too future goal oriented. If it happens, then enjoy it. It is possible to excrete urine at the same time if one has not emptied their bladder. We always use a towel on the bed, under the woman's body in any case.

There are no nerve receptors for touch on the wall of the vagina itself (think about childbirth). However, there are a lot of nerves running a little deeper than the surface and these are the areas where it feels best to stimulate.

One stroke you can do is to use two fingers inside her vagina and your thumb of that hand pushing up on the clitoral hood. These two fingers can go to whatever thunk area feels right and to stroke inside in tandem with your doing finger on her clitoris. That leaves your pinky and ring fingers of your inserted hand free to stimulate her perineum or her anus if you like and if she likes that.

A woman can have a great orgasm without any insertion. It can add to the party if done correctly but it is not necessary. Only use insertion if she really desires it and for however long she desires it. If she does not desire it then the insertion will tend to bring her down in the level of intensity she is exhibiting. In the next paragraph we will discuss how to do bring the orgasm down deliberately.

Bringing A Woman Down

Orgasm comes in all kinds of patterns. One thing that is common to all orgasms is that there is a beginning and an end, a waxing and a waning, an up cycle and a down cycle. Whether the intensity is going up or down it is all orgasmic until one has stopped feeling the sensation completely. Even an extended orgasm that has peaks that are going up for a long time will at some point tend to wane in its intensity. Every peak by definition has an upside and a downside. The difference here is that with a peak there is only a short downside and then the intensity rises again even higher.

One can deliberately take a partner down a steep slope or gradually bring someone down. It is not always necessary to bring someone down, but if she has gone high, it will definitely be beneficial to her to at least bring her down to a more comfortable state. I have found for myself and probably most guys that the down cycle is not so involved as it is for women. For men who are coming down it seems to go a lot faster compared to women, either with an ejaculation or just a had enough feeling. Of course, if a woman tensed up and went over, she would also have come down quickly just like a man does.

Intercourse is one way of bringing someone down, often for both sexes but as we have stated the intention is more important than what you are actually doing. So it is possible to go up with intercourse too. It is simple and effective to use your hands to bring a woman down. To bring a woman down from an extended relaxed orgasm the most important aspect is again to use your intention. Generally slower and firmer pressures are used. It is still your intention behind the stroke that counts most, as you can bring someone down with light quick strokes or bring someone up with firm slow ones if that is your intention.

A fun and gradual way to bring someone down is to give her peaks to create a lessoning of intensity slowly. These peaks will be probably more intense at first and progressively get less so till she reaches a level that has her feel closer to a normal state. Sometimes you may find that instead of going down she may have changed her mind and wanted some more intensity. You can tease her and take her up some more or continue to bring her down slowly. You are in control so do what feels best. Sometimes a woman will go for it the most when she thinks it is ending. Use your communication skills to find out what she is feeling. The length of these peaks will also probably get shorter and shorter on the way down. As I said she does not have to come down all the way.

One can also use heavy deliberate pressure to bring her down more quickly. Bring a woman down with a "pull-up," which is the insertion of the middle and ring finger inside her vagina. I like to use my non-doing hand to do a pull-up but you can use either hand. Put or slide your two fingers deeply inside her vagina, palm up, and pull up with pressure. At the same time press down with your second hand on the back of your inserted hand so that your palm of your inserted fingers is putting pressure on her external pelvic area. Continue with the pressure as long as it feels good to do so. You will probably feel her orgasm continue with strong contractions for a time. You can use a similar pressure with two hands pressing down on her external pelvic area if you do not wish to use any finger insertion. If your fingers are inserted, you can finish this stroke by removing them unhurriedly. Simply slide your fingers out of her vagina feeling the contact the whole way out. Once outside the vagina keep contact on her pussy with your same two fingers gently gliding up over her introitus and labia and finally sliding gently over the clitoral area. One can also use the gradual peaking on the way down method to reach a certain level and then do a pull up. Since she has already come down to some extent the pull-up will not be as dramatic.

Then you can towel her off with the washcloth that you kept nearby. You can also do this toweling off, slowly and deliberately. Some women will continue feeling and orgasming as you do this. Use whatever pressure they like best. Slow and steady is a good rule of thumb.

Sometimes women like to remain in an aroused state after getting high with orgasm. You can leave them high if this is what they want, especially if they do not have to go out and function in the world. Their state of arousal will naturally go down slowly. It will depend on how high they got and what circumstances they will encounter.

If a man has just ejaculated he will be very sensitive to any kind of touch on his penis afterwards including being toweled off. Do so very gently and slowly; more like dabbing it than rubbing with the towel. If he has not ejaculated, then he can be toweled off more gingerly as he will have less of a sensitivity of his penis.

8

Receiving Pleasure

One of the most important factors in being pleasured, if not the most important one, is to make sure that you are getting what you want and nothing unwanted is being done to you. It is not about settling for just anything although we will also soon describe how to surrender to any stroke. By getting what you want you must first know what that is. That is why it is so beneficial to experiment on yourself so that you will have some basis to guide your partner in the way of preferences. Then when you are with someone you can even before being touched communicate to them where and how you prefer to be touched.

The better one is at taking control makes it that much easier for your partner to surrender. Conversely, the better one is at surrendering their nervous system makes it that much easier for their partner to take control. Even though I get off very pleasurably I consider my real expertise is in how to pleasure a woman. Most of my writings are about that know-how. However, the art of surrendering and receiving major pleasure is just as important to our sex lives as the art of giving it. The fact is that there are many facets to controlling and giving pleasure and only a few involved to receiving it. Though there are only a few aspects to feeling immense pleasure; if you do not do them properly you will never feel the ecstasy that you are capable of. So, what are those few facets you may ask?

Being in the Moment

You will have to learn how to appreciate every moment or as many and as much of each moment with as much awareness and appreciation as you can muster. I know we have mentioned this before, but it is so vital that it bears repeating. This means that your attention is on the sensation that you are experiencing now and not on some future feeling or any other distracting thoughts. As soon as you notice that you are not focused on your feeling; put your attention back to doing so. You can repeat the short exercise from chapter 1, where you just close your eyes for a few seconds and notice any sensation in your genitals. You can do that right now.

Another practice that I learned from Eckhart Tolle in his book *The New Earth* is to feel my body, not only my genitals, as often as I can throughout the day. This will keep you grounded and is one path that he recommends to be more conscious. So, when you are in a conversation with someone or just walking along or during most anything, he suggests feeling your own body. You do not want to feel your body exclusively as you still want to listen to what someone is conversing about, or if any cars are coming to notice them of course, and so on. It is kind of like a meditation exercise that you can do anytime. I seem to feel my lips and my hands the most when I do this. I have noticed that when I am in a conversation with someone who is tumesced and talking a lot or complaining, if I put some attention on feeling my body, that it keeps me from taking on their negativity. All you must do is to feel. It is best not to compare or get into any head-trips when doing this. This is also a good practice to learn to feel more when you are being deliberately pleasured, except all or most of your attention will be on feeling your body.

Though it may seem at first to be counter-productive, communicating and approving of your pleasure will with enough practice be an asset to staying present. By verbally appreciating what is happening it allows you to be present for the following stroke, for the next moment of whatever. If you don't communicate your appreciation either you or your partner or both will be stuck on that last good stroke and not be able to focus all of your attention on the next one. We have compared it to swallowing, as you cannot keep eating if you forget to swallow the last bite you ate. By verbally acknowledging any positive sensations it will allow you to be present for the next wonderful moment.

Preferences

You must also learn your body and your preferences. That is, you want to explore what you like, where you like it and how you like to be touched. This is probably best done with self-pleasuring. It can also be done with a willing partner who you feel safe with in this exploration. If you can incorporate both of these practices, then so much the better.

The ultimate goal perhaps of surrendering your nervous system to someone other than you is to enjoy every type, every pressure, every placement and every speed that you are being touched with. I used the word perhaps because this will not be the case when you start to learn to be done. You will have preferences and it is best to honor what feels best to you. With training you will learn to stretch your envelope of what is pleasurable. You will still have preferences, but any kind of touch will be able to gratify you. We have encountered many women who really like it very lightly on their clitoris. We have also met a few who only liked it touched with a lot of pressure.

By first learning to get off really well with your preferred way of being touched you can then expand your ability to experience pleasure by adding on different touches. This does not have to be accomplished in a short time. So, if you like it lightly on your clitoris and have learned to get off well with this light stroke, keep on doing that. At some point add on a peak or just a few strokes at first with some slightly additional pressure to allow yourself to expand your limitations. Do this for only as long as it is fun and pleasurable. Practice this new addition regularly and you will develop more appreciation for it. Experiment with any new touches you can think of that are on or slightly over your boundaries of your preferences. You can widen the strike zone on your clitoris by appreciating any area that is touched. Again, start with the ones that feel the best and then add on other spots by stroking on those areas for a peak or two. By practicing you will learn to like all kinds of strokes and enjoy being touched anywhere on your clitoris.

By diligently doing the connections exercise from the self-pleasuring section you will also create new hot spots on your body that also will feel marvelous to have touched. Wherever your partner touches you or wherever you touch yourself when you desire pleasure, put all of your attention that you can on the sensation. Be greedy for as much pleasure as you can gather with as much enthusiasm as you can generate. Be focused on the stimulation that is happening at the moment. You can even have your partner do the connections exercise to you. You will have to communicate well here to strengthen any connections.

Express Yourself

Most people in our society and it is probably worse in many others are cautious and unexpressive when they are having sensual pleasure. We write about some of the things that one can voice in the communication section. Here I just want to point out that to be stingy with your appreciation will be like instant karma and the pleasure received will also be consequently reduced. Open your mouth and when it feels good, even a little good, express it out loud. It is okay to moan but to use words is a higher level of communicating. Why not do both?

When you are receiving pleasure your attention is on your feeling, on the sensation. The addition of verbalizing may at first distract you from that. Once you practice and incorporate acknowledgements into your pleasure package it will be an aid and not a hindrance. Keep it simple and short. You do not want to think deeply about what to say but just to voice what you are already feeling. The more secure you are with your rightness the less you will have to filter out.

You can even practice voicing your pleasure when self-pleasuring. Because many of us have been conditioned to not talk while having sex it will become easier with practice and over time. You don't have to scream where it wakes the neighbors. You don't want to overdo it either as that can take away from the pleasure. Most people are under expressive. Just voice how good it is and you can even connect your voice to the sensation so that it will increase your sensation. You can play with it like in a connection's exercise. Be generous with your approval and it will multiply the pleasure.

People really want to pleasure their partners. Men are valued for their ability to produce and giving their partner pleasure is one major way that a man can feel productive. If the person who is doing you is a so-called doing expert like me, don't be afraid to tell him what you like. Most guys and most people will give you what you desire. An example is simply to state what you like. So, while I am doing someone and if she would say to me, "I love the lightest and gentlest strokes the best." Then you can be sure that I would be giving her lots of gentle and the lightest strokes possible. Remember to reward your partner verbally for generating your desires.

Adding Fantasy

You can also tell a willing partner and someone you feel safe with what your favorite fantasy material is. That way they can incorporate the kind of fantasy material you like if you have any while they are pleasuring you. Not everyone likes fantasy to be used on them. Conversely not everyone will want to incorporate it into their giving of pleasure therefore I said "willing" partner. Consequently, you will have to find out. The best way is probably simply to ask if they are game. Vera for example prefers not to use any when I do her, as she just wants to feel the strokes. I like playing with fantasy and it makes it even more fun when my partner uses it when doing me.

Get It Just Right

I stated that nothing unwanted should be done to you, and you should do nothing unwanted. If your partner is doing something that does not feel good, speak up. For example, if they are using way too much pressure then tell them to do it "lighter please" or even "please a lot lighter." You can first use what I described above and just say how you love the gentlest strokes the best. If they still continue to use too much pressure you have to continue to speak up until they do it just the way you like. You can even show them on their arm with your hand how you like to be touched. You can do so before even starting or it is also perfectly fine to take a break at any time. People in general don't like to be told that they are doing something wrong. That is why it is good to use a lot of positive reinforcement along the way with plenty of approval so that they won't feel like they are letting you down. Be as polite and as nice as you can with your requests—unless it hurts—and then you must be direct. Remember to verbally acknowledge them when they respond to your preferences in a positive way.

If something actually hurts, let them know right away. Sometimes it is not even something your partner is doing but a cramp or other discomfort. Do not try to grin and bear it, as it will be almost impossible to have an orgasm under those conditions. Ask them to stop or take a break so that you can get back in the groove. You do not necessarily have to find something nice to say first. That is also why it is a good idea to build approval credit previously.

Surrender

A lot of people find it difficult to surrender their nervous system to another person. They like to stay in control and do not like to let go and relinquish what they think is their power position to someone else. The problem with this attitude is that although it might serve you elsewhere such as at work or with daily family undertakings, it is detrimental to having your optimum orgasm. You have to be vulnerable in order to have the utmost pleasure. It can be scary to be vulnerable and that is why it is difficult to be at total effect and to surrender. It is however well worth your while to develop your surrender capability.

It can be very valuable to talk to your partner before you are touched. You can explain how you like to be in control at all times but that you are working on giving it up under sensual conditions. Tell them what they can do and what they can say to have you surrender to the pleasure. This still might seem that you are controlling them to what to do and what to say but you are coaching them to what works best with you. If they are already trained, you won't have to explain too much. If they are good listeners, they will only have to be told once and then the next time that you receive pleasure from them they will know how to put you at effect and make it easier for you to surrender. Coaching is not the same as controlling. The better you are at coaching the less you will have to do it. Sometimes it will take a few times to get through to one's partner. Explain how to treat you each time as if it were the first time and do not get mad at them for not getting it as quickly as you would like.

Tell them how you prefer to be touched if they do not know this already. Everybody has their own resistances so you can get specific about yours. Teach your partner how to play with you so that you will give up your guard. I know for myself that when a woman does me, I like it when she is confident. I like it when she tells me to lay back and she is going to have her way with me. I like it when she tells me while she is stroking me that she is going to use this same stroke over and over and peak me and get close to the edge and then she is going to stop before I go over. I like it when she tells me that she can feel me in her pussy. I like it when she tells me that she can feel my contractions and that I am getting close to ejaculating. I also like to hear that she is having her own contractions as she is doing me. I like it when she reports how I am oozing or leaking all over her hand. I like it when she uses fantasy, especially about her legs and what she can do to me with them. I like it when she talks about another woman ravaging me. I like it when she tells me that she is going to take me to a place that I've never been before. I prefer not to go over at the end and will explain how to keep the peaks going. I can and have surrendered so if my partner decided to ejaculate me at the end, I am able to experience the sensation to its full extent. After the experience is over I will again explain my preferences after acknowledging the fun I just had.

This description may work for me but as I said everyone has their own likes and dislikes. Some people may like to hear that you are getting hard and turned on while stroking them and others may feel threatened by too much information of this sort. So you can let your partner know before you start what works for you. Eventually you will become more tolerant and accepting of whatever comes your way. Once you really learn to surrender it will be easy for anyone to do you and control your orgasm.

Relaxation

As we have written and taught for many years the best way to have an extended massive orgasm is to be in a relaxed state. Many women as well as most men have learned to tense up their bodies so that they can have what they think is the only way to experience an orgasm. We have demonstrated this first with our fellow orgasm explorers and then with our clients that one can learn to relax and feel way more than by tensing. We suggest that you can add on this relaxed way of coming gradually, either when you are on your own or with an untrained or even a trained lover. So, don't expect to completely switch over to being relaxed and feeling as much right away. It will probably take some time and you do not have to give up the tensing up method all together. Just consider that you are adding on a new way of feeling. It is a process.

One of the techniques that I use with some clients and that can be helpful is to switch off from tensing to being relaxed and then tensing up again and then being relaxed again. I as the doer communicate to my partner in simple terms such as "Tense your body." "Relax your body" "Tense up!" "Relax!" I will do this a bunch of times and the length of the period of each action is determined by the response. It could be only a few seconds, or it could be a couple of minutes, usually somewhere in between. Doing this exercise has several beneficial results. You can do this on your own but will be even more profitable if done with a partner. If you are the person receiving the pleasure tell your partner about this exercise so that they can take more control and give you directions.

If the woman is tensing anyhow then when I ask her to tense up I will be getting into agreement with her and therefore taking control (remember control is agreement). Then when I ask her to relax, she will automatically do that and the control will be amplified and allow her to surrender to something. You can ask your partner to play the role of control so that you can surrender your nervous system to them. I have not met anyone who resisted this exercise and argued that they wanted to keep tensing or keep relaxing. By going back and forth between these two states it also allows you to feel your body in both these conditions and how you can feel more being relaxed. You are also learning to take directions and learning to surrender your nervous system.

The same holds true when doing a guy. Even though this is a technique about giving pleasure, I thought it fit in this receiving pleasure chapter. Take control by agreement and give simple directions. Men often like to be helpful and will thrust their hips as well as active tensing, which is actually counter-productive to the pleasure of being at total effect. So, if he is doing that anyhow you can first suggest to him "thrust your hips." Now that you are in the early stages of control you can reverse that by saying, "Now relax your hips."

We had a female client who thrashed about when she was getting done, as that was the way she had always done it. By first getting her to do what she did anyway and directing her to do so we were able to take control of her nervous system and control her pleasure in a positive way. We were playful and got her to enjoy being still and feeling more.

You can even have your partner play with you if you are someone who is not feeling much by first asking you to stop feeling. Then they can say, "Feel your pussy" or "feel my hand on your clitoris." Or even "feel more" and "take it higher". You can do this with yourself too. You can have the deliberate thought to stop feeling and to start feeling and to feel it even more.

The goal is to surrender to pleasure. It is not about surrendering to an adversary as in being defeated. Your partner can learn how to take control and therefore make it easier for you to surrender. If you are both in on the game, it will be that much easier to accomplish.

Body Positions

We presented a number of different positions that one can use to do their partners manually in our previous works. We consistently like using the specific position of sitting on the bed perpendicular to your partner. That is our regular go to position for doing a woman. We advocate that the doer sits down first on the bed. Then the doer can adjust himself or herself so that they are in a comfortable state. I like to put a couple of pillows against the wall so that I can sit up against them. This way of sitting will have my back feel comfortable. Sometimes however I like to have the woman lie down first and then may play with her legs and feet and tease her genitals before joining her on the bed. I have a big towel under where I am sitting that the woman can lie down upon. I also have a pillow for her head and one to put under her outside leg. I have all my accessories nearby within arm's reach. I like to have a couple of do towels or washcloths, the lubricant and the remote for the heater and the music. Then when she lies down in a perpendicular direction to me with her head on the pillow I have her move as close to me as she can get. I have my upper leg; my right leg being that I am right-handed over her abdomen and my lower leg under her legs. Her legs are bent and are spread out as far as she can spread them without any discomfort. I place the pillow under her outside leg. My upper arm can rest and be stabilized on my bent right leg around the knee area when I am stroking her genitals. If the arm is not stabilized and is just floating in the air without any support, it will tire more easily and be less precise.

Sometimes, for certain reasons, you will have to improvise on this position. It could be because of some injury or due to either the doer or the doee being proportionately large compared to their partner. We have a friend who is in her late 60s and sometimes has a painful hip joint and also an uncomfortable area on her thigh. She has a young boyfriend who weighs around two-hundred pounds. The thigh hurts when he presses his arm or elbow against it when doing her. His leg on her pelvis area also causes her some discomfort at times. She asked us for some ideas that they can incorporate in their practice.

Vera can empathize with her as she used to say that I had bony elbows and when I touched her thigh with them it would smart. We even had one of our clients buy me some elbow pads as a joke. So, what I do now that is beneficial is to align my left forearm parallel to her thigh but press my elbow into my own leg that is placed under her legs. It is useful for support as well as that I know it is not digging into her leg. I've also used a small pillow in the past to put between my arm and her thigh. It seems the correct placing of my arm without a pillow has the same result and I can still get pleasure that way with the side of my arm touching upon her leg without the elbow being in contact. My bottom or left leg is not straight and bent as much as is necessary so that I can maneuver my hand to prop up against it also.

As far as the pressure from his leg weighing on her hips we recommended that he could kneel on the floor next to the bed. He can use as many pillows as necessary to kneel on in order to have his knees feel comfortable (one can always get knee pads) and to be at the right height. She then can lie at the edge of the bed and he can have access to her whole body and specifically her genitals. I had to use this position when I was pleasuring a large sized woman and it worked extremely well. He could also try using different size pillows on the bed under his buttocks or between his upper leg and her abdomen when in the sitting position to see if that alleviates the pressure.

It is an opportunity to be creative and you can check out these as well as create your own ways of making it more fun without the pain. Another idea is to sit in a chair next to a table like a massage table or even at the side of the bed and the woman can lie down on the table or the bed. We usually use that position with a table when we do our one-hour EMO demonstrations in front of a class. Again, it is important to stabilize the doing arm. This is often accomplished by resting it upon the woman's abdomen. I also will place a little pillow on Vera's tummy when we are in that arrangement so that I don't dig my bony elbows there either. When we are on the bed my doing or upper hand is resting on my own leg but when I am sitting next to her my arm is stabilized by resting on her abdominal area, therefore the use of the pillow.

Although this chapter is about receiving pleasure, I know I have drifted somewhat to the topic of giving pleasure. The reality is that if you know what it takes to give pleasure to yourself you can train your partner to take control of you by doing those things that will have you be at effect and allow you to surrender.

Epiloge:
Demonstration of an Extended Massive Orgasm

This description of an EMO as part of a class is a teaching tool. The following portrayal is a description of the DEMO (Demonstration of an Extended Massive Orgasm) that the young teachers performed in front of a large group of students.

Vera and I learned our basic techniques at More University in the 1970s and 80s. Vera was certified in 1980 and I was certified in 1987. Dr. Vic Baranco and Diana Goens performed the first live public demonstration in 1976 that Vera attended. Seeing the live demonstration was pivotal in Vera choosing to become a sensuality instructor. These types of demonstrations have affected many a student and so we decided to include them here in this form so perhaps we can affect some more of you. It is written in the voice of "Joseph," who is telling the story from the characters in my book *Extended Massive Orgasm: The Novel*. Although it is a fictional account it is based on participating and having attended many demonstrations.

* * *

The DEMO certifications at the end of the summer had gone beautifully. Both Keri and Maybe had the best orgasms of their lives. There was a full house of students and the show was so good that we signed a bunch of them up for personal training with the three of us and the Danboskys and Masako.

The morning session was used to get the students ready for what they would be experiencing in the afternoon. Some of the students knew only a little of the Danbosky's work and others had been studying with them for a long time, so there was a mix of experience and novices in the room. Many of the people had purchased the Danbosky's books and some of them had even read them absorbedly. The information that Saul and Joy Esther and Masako related brought the new people up to speed but was delivered in such a way that had everyone feel like they were experiencing valuable and new information. Saul told them how the best way to experience most of life's practices is with a beginner's mind. He told them how important it is for the person giving the pleasure to thoroughly enjoy what they are doing. "Have fun, be totally present and be curious," Saul continued. The same goes for you folks watching the experience. Notice what is going on and perhaps even more importantly feel the energy in the room. You can experience the orgasmic pleasure even if you are not being touched. This is easier for women than men but you all can connect with this energy."

Saul continued, "I want to do a little experiment now for one minute. I want you all to close your eyes now and put your attention on your genitals. Just feel whatever sensation you are having."

The room got quiet and I closed my eyes too. I could feel the sensation climb as more and more people got in tune with the pleasure energy that was bouncing off the walls. After Saul told them to open their eyes some of the women howled like they just had an amazing occurrence. A couple of the guys looked confused but did not say anything. Most of the women in the room had rosy cheeks and almost everyone had big grins on their faces.

One of the pretty girls sitting close to the front of the room acknowledged how she could feel her pussy as if Saul was touching it. A couple of the other women nodded in agreement. Saul then described how the afternoon would evolve, with first Keri getting certified by him. Then she would certify me and then with my certifying Maybe. He said, "Just like we all felt the energy go up a minute ago, this afternoon you will have two-plus hours of a unique opportunity to connect with the energy peaks. You can link up to the orgasm energy by just feeling your body in relation to it at any time. You will be able to feel how these energy dynamics go up and down and higher and higher.

There was time for some questions and the one I remember in particular was from a pretty young Asian woman who asked, "What is it that had you decide to have an orgasm in front of an audience?"

She was looking at Keri and Maybe and Maybe answered. "That is a great question. Orgasm is natural and beautiful. Society is so conditioned to seeing pleasure specifically orgasmic pleasure as something sinful and dirty. I am a revolutionary in that respect and want to show how positive and constructive orgasm really is. Part of becoming a teacher of orgasm includes doing it in front of others; whether it is one person at a time or a large group like this. I am also a thrill seeker and there is not much that is more thrilling than having a fantastic orgasm in front of an enthusiastic group of people. This is so much fun and what a way to make a living. Are you thinking about becoming a sensuality teacher?"

The Asian woman smiled, "This is my first time that I am being exposed to this way of thinking and it is very intriguing to me. Perhaps after I watch this afternoon, I will have a better idea but I must admit that I do like the idea."

Masako added, "You are brave for being here and being Asian like I am we have even more strong conditioning than your average person about our behavior in public so thank you so much for your question and interest."

After a lunch break, the fireworks began. Keri got certified first by Saul. He had to work if you can call that work at keeping her from getting too high too fast. The woman's job, if you can call that a job, is to feel and go as high as she can and the doers or producer of the orgasm's job is to take her for a ride and get her to where she desires to surrender her nervous system to her partner. The doer is basically using their hands to stimulate the woman's genitals and wants to keep the orgasm in a balanced and progressing movement toward higher and higher with the occasional peak thrown in to further create control and allow the woman to take the orgasm to the next level. If a person starts too high, then they can burn out too quickly.

It's kind of like riding a horse at the Kentucky derby where the horse is controlled by the jockey not to go out too fast so that they will have something left for the end of the race. Anyhow Saul took Keri for an amazing ride as he took her higher and higher with each peak. He described almost everything that he was doing to the audience and the audience was prompted to ask any questions that came up during the orgasmic celebration.

Keri was beautiful and I could tell that the audience was taking the ride with her and being present to the extended orgasm. Saul had told us before that another reason that you don't want to start too high too fast is that you can lose the audience that way. Master Light and his wife Masako first gave live and public demonstrations back in the 1970s. When they had first developed these techniques, they did not know this and started with too much intensity. The first audiences could not handle this type of powerful stimulation and would non-confront a lot of what was occurring because they could not fathom so much intensity and pleasure so quickly. People would fall asleep, space out and even a fire occurred in one of the demonstrations as people lost their awareness of the orgasm that was blasting out in front of them.

Saul began by spreading Keri's labia exposing her genitals to the class. He described what he was doing as he was doing it. He really spread the labia wide with both of his hands so that the audience could get a good view. He showed how Keri was already having contractions in the sphincter muscles, vaginally and anally as he did a little anatomy demonstration of her genitals. He told the class how he likes to look and then touch. He also said that when he is at home in the bedroom he plays with the woman's whole body before focusing in on her genitals and finally her clitoris. "It is all about the tease and getting the woman to really want to be touched." Saul related. He told them that this was a demonstration of what can be done; what is possible, not what should be done. He told them that most of the time he does not do it for so long, that twenty minutes is plenty of orgasm and you don't have to do it in a big classroom in front of many paying customers.

Saul played with Keri's pussy, deliberately not touching her clitoris. He used his knuckles in her introitus, touching her ever so gently. He lightly played with her pubic hair again arousing Keri to more sensation. He then applied the lubricant. He deliberately avoided getting any lubricant on Keri's clitoris or her clitoral hood. He moved his fingers like a musician as Buddy played a slow classical piece to accompany Saul's actions. Saul then took great pleasure in teasing Keri, gently and slowly stroking up and down her labia, one side at a time. Saul started stroking the labia closer to the clitoris with a quicker motion as Buddy increased the tempo of his accompaniment. Keri was getting higher and moaning. You could tell that Keri was aching for Saul to put his finger on her clitoris, but he was the master of tease and really had her humming.

Finally, Saul felt that Keri was completely ready and easily slipped his left hand under her buttocks and got on her spot with a bit of lubricant that Masako put on his fingertip. He accomplished both hand motions almost simultaneously similar to how a magician works on stage. Keri responded to his direct clitoral stroke and took off like a rocket ship blasting into space.

Saul was the pilot plus mission control now and showed off Keri's orgasm with numerous peaks and glorious strokes as she moaned and acknowledged him over and over with verbal appreciation. One of my favorite specific frames was when Saul took Keri down just a little bit by giving her a couple long strokes all the way to her perineum and back as Buddy finished the last song. He showed the audience how engorged Keri's clitoris was. On the first notes of the new song Saul got right back onto Keri's upper left spot and as he precisely touched her you could feel the vibrational energy of the whole room jump like tenfold. It felt like a small earthquake had penetrated my body and my hands were pulsating with sensation. A number of the students in the audience asked questions.

One young man asked, "How do you know when to start up again after you just brought her down?" Saul continued stroking as he answered. "Keri is a very responsive young woman and has been training her body for quite a while. Almost anything I do whenever I do it will work. I have no doubts and trust my feelings. She is very easy to pleasure. I don't really think about it. It just seems to flow naturally after you have been doing this for as long as I have. If she was not so accomplished the peaks would be shorter and the time between the peaks would be longer. You have to go with your gut feelings. Whenever you are pleasuring someone you want to quit him or her before they quit you. That means that you stop stroking them right before they have had enough. Then they will be in a place of wanting more and when you start to stroke them again, they will be anticipating your touch eagerly. The path to becoming a Pleasure Jedi is to practice. We recommend keeping a journal of your sensual journey. You will get better as you continue to train. Always trust your feelings and pay attention to your immediate surroundings and to your own body in bed and elsewhere. A good exercise is to be present with whatever you are doing. Whenever you find yourself head tripping somewhere else get back to the present moment. The better you are at being present and aware the better you will respond to your partner's desires." Saul kept stroking Keri as he talked. She was moaning with an abundance of ecstasy.

The guy who asked the question did not say anything, so Saul said, "That was a good question. Did I answer it to your satisfaction? It makes for better communication and makes a person a better communicator when they acknowledge any answers or responses to a question they asked or a request that was delivered that satisfies them."

"Yes! Thank you," the student sheepishly responded.

Saul kept taking Keri higher on almost every peak. She was

sustaining a high level of intensity, just coming down briefly every so often when Saul decided to do so. He continued stroking her clitoral head sometimes dancing on it to the music where he moved his finger all over Keri's clitoris. For other peaks he just stayed in her favorite pocket or favorite spot on the upper left. After about thirty minutes he started inserting his thumb of his second hand further inside Keri's vagina. When Saul first inserted his thumb, he only went in a little way like less than an inch.

This is a regular part of a DEMO and Joy Esther asked Keri, "How deep does Saul's thumb feel inside you?" Keri pointed to a spot near her belly button. Joy Esther than said to the class, "This shows that when a woman is turned on and orgasmic and relaxed her vagina is pushed out and very receptive. Penetration feels much deeper than in actuality. It also is demonstrative of the unimportance of penis size when being so receptive. A little bit can go a long way." The class had a group laugh more of a release than because Joy Esther was being funny. It was quite the show.

Saul was pleased with his handiwork and Keri's orgasmic certainty and certified her after forty minutes or so of orgasmic ascension. He turned her over to me at that point. People had been continually asking questions to both Saul and Keri, which they were able to handle with ease. Strangely, I was not nervous at all. I jumped right in as if I had been pleasuring women in front of a class for my whole life. I felt calm and at ease at the controls and Keri was ready to go into the final stretch with lots of passion and desire for even more sensation. Her clitoris was totally exposed, and she was so easy to pleasure. I explained how the last 30 minutes of the demonstration is where penetration with the second hand into the vagina is possible. Saul had already been playing with both of his hands for the past ten minutes and when I took over the two fingers (index and middle fingers) of my bottom hand were immediately sucked into Keri's vagina almost like a vacuum cleaner with strong suction.

I stroked her G-spot area with these two fingers in a come-hither motion, as I stroked her clitoris with short precise strokes on her upper left quadrant with the index finger of my upper hand—very simple and easy. Keri went up higher with each stroke and her vagina was totally wet and luscious to feel. Her clitoris was bulbous and a deep red color. I could hear her soft moans with each stroke, and I could sense the folks especially the women in the audience feel the strokes as if I was doing it to them. This was bliss. My brother Buddy was making these beautiful notes on the guitar that harmonized with the tactile sensation that I was feeling. It was like the electronic waves of the music and the electricity from Keri's pussy met for an instant and combined into a giant wave of increasing sensation that filled my body and everyone else in the room with this raw feeling of exploration and ecstasy.

I skipped a beat and Buddy did the same at the exact moment as we temporarily gave ourselves a breath to exhale and allow the orgasm and the movement to take off again for another peak. That moment of not touching and of no music is also of blissful and what creates the next first stroke and first note to be noticed as a majestic beauty, which is exactly what I felt when I put my finger back on that amazing clitoris.

Then the parade of students began as Saul allowed them one at a time to come up to the front of the room and put their hand on Keri's upper thigh. He split the room in two as there were over fifth students in attendance, too many to have come up in one show. Saul told them that half the room or side A would come up now and touch Keri and the other half or side B could have the chance to come up when Maybe would be having her orgasm.

Besides putting their hand on Keri's thigh I offered some of them to position their other hand on Keri's abdomen so they could feel her abdominal ridging. Most of the women were able to feel a lot of the sensation in their own pussy when they physically connected with Keri. I would take her on a peak and they would come along for the ride. Each person who came up to touch Keri got a personal peak. When Tiffany came up, I teased her, saying that she would be up here soon. She got me back by getting me hard, which is a nice way to be gotten back at, and Tiffany and Keri really went high together. A specific frame was when Keri ejaculated on my penetrating hand and onto the table as I was massaging her G-Spot area. My finger on her clitoris felt like a hero who had single handedly won the war and was being appreciated as if her clitoris was stroking my finger instead of me stroking her.

Saul said, "That was fun Keri. She just had an ejaculation. Did you all see that?" About half of the class answered that they had, the other half remaining quiet. Saul continued, "Keri does not ejaculate every time and it really is not something to strive for. It is fun when it does, and it makes for a good show. There are some glands associated with the G-Spot that release the ejaculate into her urethra and that is where the ejaculate is excreted and squirted. There are other glands in a woman's vagina that release vaginal fluids that can vary in consistency from very thick to less so. These are not squirted out like you just saw but kind of ooze out of a woman who is being stimulated and aroused. It is not something to strive for either, but notice it when it does occur."

After the peak and a short break I had fun when Kadija, when the girl from the boutique, came up to put her hand on Keri. I made sure that she could feel and connect with the orgasm. I took Keri on the highest peak so far where the sensation on my fingertip felt as if it were one with Keri's clitoris. Being part of Keri at this point I could feel this giant oceanic wave with tremendous energy crash onto the side of the island.

A whole slew of folks took advantage of this opportunity to enjoy Keri's waves and Keri and I gave each one of them a marvelous ride. We then did the group connection where everyone held hands. Saul was on one side holding Keri's foot and Joy Esther was holding her other foot, reaching out with their other hand to someone in the audience. Saul then had everyone close their eyes and feel the sensation go through them. I gave Keri some sensational strokes on her spot and she went for the highest amount of sensation using the connection of the room to ramp up her orgasm to a new level of awareness. My finger felt like it fit perfectly in that sexy pocket at the top left side of Keri's clitoris as if held in place by a magnetic field. The sensation jumped and my own body awareness jumped too, so that I felt totally alive with joy and love. It felt like we were all hovering above the ground in a spiritual amusement ride. After that group orgasm, Saul, Joy Esther and Masako announced that I was certified with honors.

They had me bring Keri down which I did as best I could, as she was so high it would probably take days if ever to fully come back to how she was before starting. I gave her some short peaks on the way down with some heavy pressure with pull-ups and body pressure. I wiped her off and then gave her a solid kiss on her lips as she sat up and faced the audience. They were all cheering her for a great performance. It was encore time for me, and next up was Maybe.

We took a short break to allow folks to stretch their legs and to come back to earth so that they could confront and enjoy the second act. The Danboskys and Masako and Keri and Maybe and I all got together in the back room where we hugged Keri like crazy. Saul and Joy and Masako were very approving and happy. When everyone was reseated, we reentered the room. The room despite the break was still high from Keri's orgasm. I took off Maybe's robe. She was wearing the golden one I gave her in Rome.

She lay down on the table and I started feeling her body with my hand hovering a few inches away from her skin. The energy coming off her body felt like it was sparkling bubbles with a twist of light. It felt similar to the sensation I get when I place my hand over a glass of soda pop. As I moved my hand around her body the energy would be stronger and warmer and felt thicker near her genitals. I then touched her skin starting with those favorite sexy thighs of Maybe's that so enchanted me. I stroked her with light sensual touches circling around her thighs, first her left thigh and then her right one. She was in orgasm already and I did not want her to go up too fast and I backed off and gave her some firmer stokes around her shoulders and upper arms. It was fun touching those areas too, just not quite as sensational. I moved my hands to her abdomen and did some light circles there too. I went back to Maybe's thighs and did some up and down strokes on the inner part. Maybe started moaning and I could feel my crotch respond to her pleasure. I could feel the audience being enthralled with Maybe's orgasm already as they were all focused on her crotch. I lightly danced over her pubic hair for one second and I could feel her intensity increase. I told the audience that I was going to do a quick anatomy demonstration. I put one hand on each side of her outer labia and spread her labia apart to expose her female erotic region. Her contractions were strongly visible, and I pointed them out to everyone. Someone asked if she was doing that voluntarily and Maybe said, "No way."

I pointed out her perineum, introitus and how the top of her inner labia met at the base of her clitoris. I pulled back the hood of her clitoris by pressing my palm slightly above it toward her body and in an up direction. The hood moved away easily exposing her gorgeous clitoris, which was of a beautiful soft pinkish color. I then played with her public hair some more showing how much sensation one can have just doing that. Masako gave me some lubrication on my hand and I gently put some on Maybe's perineum, moving my finger around the area in a circular motion. I could sense Maybe feeling the pleasure of my stroke there so continued touching her there for a little longer. Masako then gave me some more lubricant on my index and middle finger. I lubricated Maybe's inner labia with one finger on either labium at the same time. I went slowly up and down her labia as Maybe continued to moan with joy. I then went to my index finger, only stroking the right labia and then switching to the left one. I was stroking them gently with an up and down movement, all the way up and all the away down without removing my finger except when I switched labia. The upper part of Maybe's labia especially on the left side was sensitive and responsive to my touch. She was getting higher each time I touched that area. I decided to play for a while in this area with light little quick caresses that Maybe once had described as butterfly wing strokes. Maybe was having her first big peak before I even stroked her directly on her clitoris. Maybe did not have to wait much longer as it was time to do some bread-and-butter strokes on her upper left quadrant.

I placed my left hand under Maybe's luscious buttocks with my thumb firmly but not penetrating against the bottom of her introitus. Maybe felt so wonderful in my hands. I could feel her orgasm as electric sensation tickling my hands and entering down my arms into my body. The sensation of her skin against my hands and arms was such a friendly felling like coming back home after a long journey. She had deliciously smooth cheeks and her pussy was engorging and wet.

I hooked the index finger of my right orgasm engendering hand smack into that succulent and eagerly awaiting pocket at the top left of her clitoris. The orgasm jumped higher as I started my rhythmical stroking as Buddy played along enhancing the experience. I started off using light pressure with a medium speed and a very short up and down movement like those little butterfly wings again staying in that pocket without leaving. I continued the exact same stroke acknowledging to Maybe as to how much pleasure I was receiving from touching her. Maybe was also acknowledging my touches with lots of approval.

Maybe said, "Yes, that is perfect. I was anticipating you touching me right there. You have fantastic magical fingers, Joseph. You are right on my spot. This feels amazing."

I kept doing the same stroke for a few minutes, as Maybe's orgasm grew more intense and sensational. She had surrendered her nervous system and whatever I did now she would respond with enthusiastic pleasure. Someone in the audience asked, "How do you know when to change the stroke and peak her?"

I spoke to the class as I continued to stroke in that exquisite pocket. "I am doing what feels good to me. It should feel easy and the simpler the better. As soon as the next stroke does not feel as good as the previous one will remind me to change the stroke. When I am in tune with Maybe I know that even before it happens, so I just stop or change when I feel the inkling, like now," as I took my hand off and showed the class how engorged Maybe's clitoris had become. I then put my finger back on her spot and continued, perhaps a little quicker stroke this time. "You see, once she surrenders it does not really matter the exact second that I peak her as she will allow me to control her orgasm without any resistance. She trusts that I will do right by her and I will. The better one is at giving pleasure the easier it is for your partner to surrender and the better your partner is at receiving pleasure, the easier it is to take control of that orgasm."

Someone in the audience then asked, "How do you know when to put your finger back on?"

"It's like Saul said. You have to trust in yourself and have confidence in your feelings. Once your partner surrenders like Maybe has, it really does not matter what you do. I can take my hand off or play with her labia or do whatever I feel like and she will follow the pleasure," as I took my hand off again and played with Maybe's labia and wet introitus. "The orgasm has lost only a little in intensity now while I am playing south of her clitoris. Maybe has given me a big strike zone so wherever I put my finger she will enjoy it to the fullest. When I feel like taking her on another intense peak, I can use my intention and start stroking purposefully to bring the orgasm higher," which I did by putting my finger back on her spot and using short quick strokes that had Maybe moaning with intense ecstasy.

The questioners had learned something from Saul as they all acknowledged that we had answered their questions even though some of these questions were already asked and answered previously.

"What does it feel like to you, Maybe, when Joseph puts his finger back on your spot? Does it feel different than what he was doing before?"

I slowed down the speed of the stroke a little so Maybe could answer the question. "I am putting my energy into feeling whatever sensation I can. I am in complete feeling mode. It's being fully present. I can feel Joseph's intention to take me higher, but I don't think about it. I just react to what he is doing, and my body just responds with the intensity level building and the pleasure feeling increasing. It feels better and better."

I said, "How many people can feel their own body's orgasm in relation to Maybe's?" About half of the woman raised their hands including Masako and Esther. "That is great," I said. "Now I want everyone to put their attention on their own genitals and just feel the orgasm that is filling the room.

Masako said, "That's better; I can feel almost every woman now and even a couple of the guys going for it."

"You see", Saul said. "Orgasm is really easy. All you have to do is have your attention on it and it will be there."

The story continues!

Acknowledgements

Even though I have never met these spiritual teachers I am so grateful to have had the opportunity to read their books. The list includes Eckhart Tolle, Frank Kinslow, Jon Kabat-Zinn, Elizabeth Gilbert and Joshua *aka* Jesus Christ. They have taught me how to be more patient, more loving and more accepting of all the curve balls that life throws at you.

I am forever grateful to Dr. Vic Baranco and the Morehouse or at times More University group who have paved the way for my ride through the Looking Glass of Orgasm and Pleasure.

I have taken this ride with my Captain and pilot Vera Bodansky who is my muse, my mojo, and my magic.

I am very grateful to Dr. Christiane Northrup who is out there in the world generating more love and kindness. Wherever she goes and whomever she touches becomes a better human being. I really appreciate all the kind words that she has consistently said about our work.

I am thrilled to have met and participated along with Vera in Heather Graham's first screenplay and directorial debut in the movie Half Magic. She was so nice to let us sit in her director's seat to watch some of the filming. Although the editor deleted that story from this book and the producer deleted our scene from the movie, I am still awed by the experience.

I truly appreciated the kindness and friendliness that Molly Shannon showed us on the movie-set. It made our experience in LA more memorable and more fun.

I am so pleased to have met good friends while I was writing this book. They all had their own part to play in helping me create this manuscript. Chad Cameron, Kristina Cooper and George Wiel. Chad helped me get my iMac in running shape with a newer version of Microsoft word than I was using before. He also initiated getting our DVD available as a download and helped us with a number of techno questions that I bumped up against. He also shares my passion for creative ideas. Kristina is a lovely young woman who was kind enough to donate her pussy for some of the research that I was doing while creating new strokes. She also brings the intensity level of Chad to a more human level. George is also a computer whiz and enabled me to continue whenever I was technologically stuck. Sometimes I would figure out the answer while just composing the question to him. He is that talented.

I appreciate Bruce Thomashauer for his continued friendship and that he is willing to listen to my bullshit and my brilliant insights at almost any time of the day.

I would also like to thank Vladimir who has more questions than the show *Jeopardy*. His questions are always food for thought.

I am grateful to know Frank Borreani who is a good friend and fellow voyager.

I am grateful to Marc Benetau who posed the idea of the video about "A Do Date", which turned out to be the chapter on overcoming resistances.

I am grateful for Marlene who takes such wonderful care of my mom along with her sister Lorna.

I am impressed and appreciate my fellow traveler Betsy Blankenbaker for the courage that she has demonstrated in her life and in her autobiography of her Orgasm.

Acknowledgements

I am forever grateful to our friend Regena Thomashauer who is out there publicly in front of the world bravely and delightfully espousing women to more pleasure.

I am extremely grateful to Maryann Karinch, my agent, editor and publisher for having the faith in me and giving this book the opportunity to be realized.

Most of all I am grateful to you dear reader for your enjoyment in our work.

Bibliography

Baranco, Vic. *I Dogma: Vol. 1.* More University Press, 1986.

Blankenbaker, Betsy. *Autobiography of an Orgasm.* 2014.

Bodansky, Vera and Steve. *Extended Massive Orgasm.* Alameda, CA: Hunter House Publishers, 2000

Bodansky, Vera and Steve. *The Illustrated Guide to Extended Massive Orgasm.* Alameda, CA: Hunter House Publishers, 2002.

Bodansky, Vera and Steve. *To Bed or Not To Bed: What Men Want, What Women Want, How Great Sex Happens.* Alameda, CA: Hunter House Publishers, 2006.

Bodansky, Vera and Steve. *Instant Orgasm: Excitement at First Touch:* Alameda, CA: Hunter House Publishers, 2008.

Bodansky, Steve. *Extended Massive Orgasm: The Novel.* Walnut Creek, California: self, 2013.

Bodansky, Steve. Switch Pitcher: Evolution of Darwin: Walnut Creek, California: self, 2015.

Bodansky, Steve. *Love and Alzheimer's:* Walnut Creek, California: self, 2018

Fisher, Helen. *The Sex Contract: The Evolution of Human Behavior*. New York, NY: William Morrow, 1982.

Gilbert, Elizabeth. *Big Magic: Creative Living Beyond Fear*. New York, NY: Riverhead Books, 2015

Kinslow, Frank. *The Kinslow System: Your Path to Proven success in Heath, Love, and Life*. USA: Hay House Inc. 2013.

Last, Walter. *The Neurochemistry of Sex*. Internet, 2011.

Lynne, Ginger. *On Blossoming: Frank and Practical Advice on Our bodies, Sexual Health, Sensuality, Pleasure, Orgasm, and More*: New York, NY: Skyhorse Publishing, 2019.

Thomashauer, Regena. *Mamagena's School for Womanly Arts: Using the Power of Pleasure to Have Your Way with the World*. New York, NY: Simon and Schuster, 2002.

Tolle, Eckhart. *The Power of Now*. Namaste Publishing, 2004.

Tolle, Eckhart. *A New Earth: Awakening to your Life's Purpose*. New York, NY: the Penguin Group, 2005.

Wallen, Kim and Lloyd, Elizabeth. *Female Sexual Arousal: Genital Anatomy and Orgasm in Intercourse*. Internet, 2011

Weeks, David. *Sex is the secret to Looking Younger*. Internet, 2013.

Whipple, Beverly and Komisaruk, Barry. *The Orgasm Answer Guide*. Johns Hopkins University Press, 2009

Zinn, Jon Kabat. Mindfulness for Beginners: Reclaiming the Present Moment--and Your Life. Louisville, Colorado: Sounds True Publishers, 2006

Author Biography

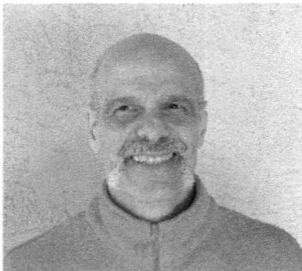

Steve Bodansky and his wife Vera have been teachers of sensuality for the past 35 years. Steve received a Masters in Molecular Genetics at SUNY at Albany and a Doctorate at More University in sensuality with an emphasis on female orgasm. He first studied and then taught at More University through 1992. For the past thirty years, they have been coaching students to expand their orgasmic potential and to improve their relationships. A number of their former students have become sensual facilitators themselves. Steve has written numerous books about optimizing sensual pleasure, including two best sellers: *Extended Massive Orgasm* and *The Illustrated Guide to Extended Massive Orgasm.*

Also by Steve and Vera Bodansky

Extended Massive Orgasm
The Illustrated Guide to Extended Massive Orgasm
Instant Orgasm
To Bed or Not to Bed
Extended Massive Life: A True Love Story and More
Extended Massive Orgasm: The Novel
Pigetry
Universe of Love
Switch Pitcher: Evolution of Darwin
Love and Alzheimer's
Orbit: Looking for Libido